A Healthcare Provider's Guide to Cancer and Obesity

Anne Katz, PhD, RN, FAAN

Oncology Nursing Society
Pittsburgh, Pennsylvania

ONS Publications Department
Publisher and Director of Publications: William A. Tony, BA, CQIA
Managing Editor: Lisa M. George, BA
Assistant Managing Editor: Amy Nicoletti, BA, JD
Acquisitions Editor: John Zaphyr, BA, MEd
Copy Editors: Vanessa Kattouf, BA, Andrew Petyak, BA
Graphic Designer: Dany Sjoen
Editorial Assistant: Judy Holmes

Library of Congress Cataloging-in-Publication Data
Names: Katz, Anne (Anne Jennifer), 1958- author. | Oncology Nursing Society, issuing body.
Title: A healthcare provider's guide to cancer and obesity / Anne Katz.
Other titles: Guide to cancer and obesity
Description: Pittsburgh, Pennsylvania : Oncology Nursing Society, [2017] | Includes bibliographical references and index.
Identifiers: LCCN 2016052624 | ISBN 9781935864943 (paperback)
Subjects: | MESH: Neoplasms--etiology | Neoplasms--prevention & control | Obesity--complications | Weight Reduction Programs--methods | Body Weight Maintenance | Motivational Interviewing
Classification: LCC RC261 | NLM QZ 202 | DDC 616.99/4--dc23 LC record available at https://lccn.loc.gov/2016052624

Publisher's Note

This book is published by the Oncology Nursing Society (ONS). ONS neither represents nor guarantees that the practices described herein will, if followed, ensure safe and effective patient care. The recommendations contained in this book reflect ONS's judgment regarding the state of general knowledge and practice in the field as of the date of publication. The recommendations may not be appropriate for use in all circumstances. Those who use this book should make their own determinations regarding specific safe and appropriate patient care practices, taking into account the personnel, equipment, and practices available at the hospital or other facility at which they are located. The author and publisher cannot be held responsible for any liability incurred as a consequence from the use or application of any of the contents of this book. Figures and tables are used as examples only. They are not meant to be all-inclusive, nor do they represent endorsement of any particular institution by ONS. Mention of specific products and opinions related to those products do not indicate or imply endorsement by ONS. Websites mentioned are provided for information only; the hosts are responsible for their own content and availability. Unless otherwise indicated, dollar amounts reflect U.S. dollars.

ONS publications are originally published in English. Publishers wishing to translate ONS publications must contact ONS about licensing arrangements. ONS publications cannot be translated without obtaining written permission from ONS. (Individual tables and figures that are reprinted or adapted require additional permission from the original source.) Because translations from English may not always be accurate or precise, ONS disclaims any responsibility for inaccuracies in words or meaning that may occur as a result of the translation. Readers relying on precise information should check the original English version.

Printed in the United States of America

ONS®
Oncology Nursing Society

Innovation • Excellence • Advocacy

Writing a book is, for the most part, a solitary endeavor, but people are always in the wings who read and review, comment and suggest, and, ultimately, make the work better in process and end product. I could not even begin to think about writing without the support, encouragement, critique, and suggestions of my husband, Dr. Alan Katz, who makes just about everything better.

Disclosure

Editors and authors of books and guidelines provided by the Oncology Nursing Society are expected to disclose to the readers any significant financial interest or other relationships with the manufacturer(s) of any commercial products.

A vested interest may be considered to exist if a contributor is affiliated with or has a financial interest in commercial organizations that may have a direct or indirect interest in the subject matter. A "financial interest" may include, but is not limited to, being a shareholder in the organization; being an employee of the commercial organization; serving on an organization's speakers bureau; or receiving research funding from the organization. An "affiliation" may be holding a position on an advisory board or some other role of benefit to the commercial organization. Vested interest statements appear in the front matter for each publication.

Contributors are expected to disclose any unlabeled or investigational use of products discussed in their content. This information is acknowledged solely for the information of the readers.

The author provided the following disclosure and vested interest information:

The author had no relevant information to disclose.

Contents

Preface

It seems that every day there is something in the news, on television, and reported in the literature about the role that obesity plays in the development of one disease or another. This is true for cancer, too, and it is often difficult to keep up with the seemingly constant evidence that is being reported.

The evidence for the link between obesity and cancer is clear and strong: obesity is linked to the development of certain cancers and to recurrence in others. Obesity is a modifiable risk factor but one that is challenging to modify. It is also a topic that is often difficult to talk about—and not just between friends and family members. Healthcare providers also find it difficult to talk about. Some of us refuse to raise the topic with our patients despite the evidence that it is important to talk about it and that our patients find it acceptable and perhaps even encouraging. Many healthcare providers struggle with the same issues as our patients. We may have gained weight over the years and have not managed to do anything about it. Some of us have tried to lose weight over and over and over again, only to see the pounds and inches creep back on. I often hear my colleagues say that they cannot tell a patient to lose weight because they themselves are overweight or obese. I see that as a bridge to the patient. Admitting that we, too, have fought the battle of the bulge and lost is a way of connecting, of admitting that it is difficult and that we understand their situation.

Many of us have had to tell our patients that they are at risk for disease or have had to convey the devastating news of a cancer diagnosis. Patients and their partners or families will often ask, "Is there anything we can do to make a difference?" They are looking for something tangible they can do to alter the course of the disease. We can talk about emotional and instrumental support and monitoring for symptoms, but this is also a golden opportunity to talk about the lifestyle changes that may make a very real difference in the outcomes for our patients. Controlling what we eat is a challenge for many people. Some of us eat to live while others live to eat. Some of us love to exercise while others would rather walk on hot coals.

Changing how and what we eat and making time for exercise can seem daunting in the face of cancer treatment. However, it can help on so many levels. As healthcare providers, we have a responsibility to help our patients help themselves. This does not mean expecting behavior change but giving patients the tools to make changes, should they choose to do so.

This book is an effort to remove the taboo around this sensitive topic. It is not intended to make the reader an expert in nutrition or exercise; we have colleagues who are the experts in these areas. The primary focus of this book is on having the conversation, finding the words, breaking down the barriers, and enlightening our patients that there is something they can do in the face of cancer that will improve their lives, decrease their risk of recurrence and poor outcomes, and, if their families join them, reduce their loved ones' risk of developing cancer in some instances.

Chapter 1
Introduction

Overweight and obesity are significant factors in the incidence of acute and chronic health conditions, including cancer. The American Society of Clinical Oncology (ASCO) recognizes the significance of the role that overweight and obesity plays in the risk for the development of certain cancers as well as the increased risk of recurrence and poor outcomes for cancer survivors (Ligibel et al., 2014). Systemic chemotherapy for overweight and obese patients may be given at subtherapeutic doses because of concerns about toxicity with doses that are based on the actual weight of patients (Lyman & Sparreboom, 2013); this can result in suboptimal response to treatment.

The Centers for Disease Control and Prevention suggest a tipping point has been reached where advances in the treatment of diseases no longer compensate for the contribution of overweight and obesity to the development of chronic diseases (Ludwig, 2016). Obesity-related cancers are now recognized as an accepted definition for certain cancers, such as breast, prostate, endometrial, and kidney. Evidence is likely to emerge that other rare cancers are similarly related to overweight and obesity (Azvolinsky, 2014).

The mechanisms for this increased risk of obesity-related cancers are multifactorial; however, overweight and obesity are preventable. They do not require expensive interventions to control, but weight management is challenging.

ASCO recommends that all patients with cancer be weighed and their body mass index (BMI) calculated (see Chapter 11). Based on their weight and BMI, patients should be advised whether they need to lose weight or prevent weight gain. They should be encouraged to eat a healthy diet and to incorporate physical activity into their daily lives to both improve quality of life and decrease the incidence of comorbidity. Patients should be referred to specialist services such as nutritionists, exercise physiologists, and rehabilitation specialists as needed to help them in this endeavor (Ligibel et al., 2014).

Despite their knowledge of the risks of being overweight or obese and their desire to improve their overall health, cancer survivors do not necessarily make the appropriate modifications to their diet and activity level. In fact, one study showed that cancer survivors do not adhere to the guidelines for a healthy diet recommended by the U.S. Department of Agriculture's 2010 *Dietary Guidelines for Americans* (Zhang, Liu, John,

Must, & Demark-Wahnefried, 2015). Patients want more information about diet, physical activity, and weight management, but their oncology care providers may not be providing them with the information they need (James-Martin, Koczwara, Smith, & Miller, 2014). Talking to patients about their weight and the need to lose weight is a topic that often is fraught with tension for both healthcare providers and patients. To date, very little data exist on the role that oncology care providers play in counseling patients about how excess weight affects morbidity and mortality. However, it is recognized that oncology care providers have an important role in educating patients.

Overview of Chapters

The first five chapters in this book describe what we know about cancer and obesity, nutritional recommendations, and physical activity in the context of cancer survivorship. This is a growing field of research, with new discoveries and evidence being published on a regular basis. The next five chapters contain information about the psychosocial aspects of weight management, including practical guidance on how to motivate, encourage, and assist survivors to lose weight and increase their physical activity. This section also contains information on the barriers to lifestyle change and how to help patients who face challenges in their attempts to do so. The final chapter contains useful resources for healthcare providers, including guidelines and websites that can support practice in this area.

Chapter 2. Overweight and Obesity and the Risk of Cancer and Poor Outcomes

This chapter describes how overweight and obesity are linked to the risk of developing cancer and the increased risk of recurrence or poor outcomes, including death.

Chapter 3. Weight Management

This chapter describes the most common and popular approaches to weight loss and presents evidence on weight loss in noncancer populations. Very little data on this topic exist for cancer populations. This is partly because undesirable weight loss has been the most common issue for many patients with cancer, and most studies focus on prevention and management of cachexia. However, given the increasing evidence on the role of overweight and obesity as risk factors for cancer and cancer recurrence, attention should be paid to weight loss in overweight or obese cancer survivors and how best to encourage weight loss where appropriate.

Chapter 4. Optimal Nutrition

This chapter presents what we know about optimal nutrition for cancer survivors. Oncology care providers need to know the evidence about these claims and advice to guide and educate their patients to eat as well as possible to both lose weight and maintain a healthy weight to promote healing from treatment and overall good health.

Chapter 5. Physical Activity and Weight Management

This chapter describes research on physical activity and body weight and programs and interventions that focus on exercise and weight loss. The chapter addresses how individuals can increase their motivation to incorporate physical activity and exercise in their daily life and includes suggestions for oncology care providers to assist patients and survivors in integrating physical activity and exercise into their lives.

Chapter 6. Barriers and Facilitators to Lifestyle Change

This chapter describes the evidence about lifestyle changes for cancer survivors, with an emphasis on breast, prostate, and colorectal cancers. Much of the research describes the barriers and facilitators to lifestyle change as identified by cancer survivors and their oncology team.

Chapter 7. Communicating About Weight Issues With Patients

This chapter describes the challenges that we as oncology care providers have in discussing weight-related issues with our patients and among ourselves. It provides the reader with a toolkit of resources to initiate the conversation and to offer assistance to patients. It also addresses the sensitive issue of personal weight in healthcare providers and how it affects our willingness or refusal to discuss this topic with our patients.

Chapter 8. Motivational Interviewing

This chapter explains the basic tenets of motivational interviewing and suggests how oncology care providers can use this technique to involve patients in the decisions needed to both accept and change attitudes and behaviors contributing to overweight and obesity.

Chapter 9. Mindfulness and Overweight and Obesity

This chapter provides a brief overview of mindfulness and how it is used in reducing physical and psychological effects of illness, including cancer. The evidence on mindfulness-based interventions targeting weight control is described, and resources for providers and patients are listed at the end of the chapter. Related topics, including intuitive and mindful eating, are briefly discussed.

Chapter 10. Challenges Faced by Patients Who Want to Lose Weight

This chapter highlights what oncology care providers need to know and understand about why it is so difficult for patients to do what seems best for themselves in this area—in part to be able to help patients overcome these barriers and also in an effort to support them through this challenging time. This chapter also addresses how care providers can handle patients who do not want to make the beneficial lifestyle changes necessary to lose weight.

Chapter 11. Resources

This chapter highlights a number of resources for oncology care providers and other healthcare providers that offer guidance and assistance for those who want to learn more about managing overweight and obesity in their patients. Guidelines specific to cancer care in the context of overweight and obesity are beginning to be developed and are presented in this chapter.

What This Book Provides

This book outlines the evidence for encouraging patients who are overweight or obese to make the necessary lifestyle changes to maximize their health and prevent recurrence of primary disease and the development of a secondary cancers, mitigate side effects, and potentiate optimal recovery from treatment and return to health after treatment. Each chapter presents what is known about the various topics as well as case vignettes with questions to prompt discussion and encourage reflection about practice. Examples also are given on ways to discuss weight management and physical activity with patients. The intent is to educate oncology care providers about the extant evidence about cancer and overweight and obesity, recognizing that this is an evolving field. It also is intended to provide oncology care providers with the tools and resources to talk to their patients about overweight and obesity to encourage and promote behavior change and reduce the risks conferred by these phenomena.

References

Azvolinsky, A. (2014). Cancer risk: The fat tissue–BMI–obesity connection. *Journal of the National Cancer Institute, 106*(4), 4–6. doi:10.1093/jnci/dju100

James-Martin, G., Koczwara, B., Smith, E.L., & Miller, M.D. (2014). Information needs of cancer patients and survivors regarding diet, exercise and weight management: A qualitative study. *European Journal of Cancer Care, 23,* 340–348. doi:10.1111/ecc.12159

Ligibel, J.A., Alfano, C.M., Courneya, K.S., Demark-Wahnefried, W., Burger, R.A., Chlebowski, R.T., … Hudis, C.A. (2014). American Society of Clinical Oncology position statement on obesity and cancer. *Journal of Clinical Oncology, 32,* 3568–3574. doi:10.1200/JCO.2014.58.4680

Ludwig, D.S. (2016). Lifespan weighed down by diet. *JAMA, 315,* 2269–2270. doi:10.1001/jama.2016.3829

Lyman, G.H., & Sparreboom, A. (2013). Chemotherapy dosing in overweight and obese patients with cancer. *Nature Reviews Clinical Oncology, 10,* 451–459. doi:10.1038/nrclinonc.2013.108

Zhang, F.F., Liu, S., John, E.M., Must, A., & Demark-Wahnefried, W. (2015). Diet quality of cancer survivors and noncancer individuals: Results from a national survey. *Cancer, 121,* 4212–4221. doi:10.1002/cncr.29488

Chapter 2

Overweight and Obesity and the Risk of Cancer and Poor Outcomes

The association between overweight and obesity and cancer has become clearer over the past decades, with growing evidence linking the two in the development of certain cancers, the risk of recurrence, and the increase in morbidity and mortality. Cancers of the breast, endometrium, prostate, and kidney, as well as colorectal cancer, are all associated with weight, body mass index (BMI), waist-to-height ratio, waist-to-hip ratio (WHR), weight-to-height ratio, and waist circumference (Heo et al., 2015).

This field is ripe for research, both bench and applied, and is an area in which health promotion in all individuals, whether they have been diagnosed with cancer or not, can be applied. This chapter will describe how overweight and obesity are linked to the risk of developing cancer and the increased risk of recurrence or poor outcomes, including death.

Development of Cancer

Breast Cancer

The role of overweight and obesity in the risk for and development of breast cancer is the most articulated in the literature to date. It is well established that women with breast cancer gain weight (Vance, Mourtzakis, McCargar, & Hanning, 2011); this is particularly true for premenopausal women and those who receive chemotherapy of longer duration. Even those women whose weight remains stable during treatment are known to gain weight over the ensuing years. Being overweight or obese, often referred to as "having greater adiposity" (Chan & Norat, 2015), is a risk factor for a number of adverse events, including risk of recurrence, death, secondary cancers, poor quality of life, and the development of lymphoma (Chlebowski, Aiello, & McTiernan, 2002; Druesne-Pecollo et al., 2012; Montazeri, 2008; Niraula, Ocana, Ennis, & Goodwin, 2012; Protani, Coory, & Martin, 2010; Velanovich & Szymanski, 1999).

In addition, overweight and obesity predisposes women to cardiovascular disease, diabetes, and hypertension, all of which can shorten life span and negatively affect quality of life. Obese women may not receive the optimal dose of chemotherapy because total dose may not be calculated according to their BMI but rather on their body surface area; this may result in less than optimal treatment outcomes as compared to women of normal weight (Fontanella et al., 2015). Obese women may be more difficult to diagnose due to larger breast size and may eventually be found to have larger tumor size, more aggressive disease, and disease that is estrogen receptor (ER), progesterone receptor, and HER2 negative, all of which suggest a poor prognosis (Copson et al., 2015). In this study of premenopausal women with breast cancer, overall survival and distant disease-free interval were lower in obese patients compared to those of normal weight at eight years after diagnosis.

The link between breast cancer and overweight and obesity is proposed to be related to elevated levels of estrogen as a result of aromatization of androgens to estrogens in adipose tissue. Estrogen promotes cell proliferation, and this is found particularly in hormone-sensitive breast cancers (Cleary & Grossman, 2009). Androgens also may be implicated in breast cancer, although their role is not clear at this time. It is thought that some of the risk factors for breast cancer, such as obesity, may result in higher estrogen levels due to aromatization of testosterone in fatty tissue (Zhang et al., 2015).

Evidence exists that ethnicity may play a role in the development of breast cancer. For example, breast cancer in African American women is dependent on menopausal status and subtype of breast cancer (ER positive or ER negative). Bandera et al. (2015) found that higher BMI in postmenopausal women was associated with increased risk for ER-positive breast cancer, while high BMI in young adults was associated with a decreased risk of ER-positive disease. This study also found that the risk for triple-negative breast cancer was elevated in women with central obesity, suggesting that this subtype of breast cancer may be more strongly associated with metabolic syndrome comprising central obesity, insulin resistance, dyslipidemia, and hypertension than with estrogen.

Others have supported the role of cardiometabolic factors in the development of breast cancer. *Metabolic syndrome* is defined as three of the following five factors: central obesity, hypertension, low high-density lipoprotein (HDL) cholesterol, high blood glucose, and high triglyceride levels. In a study of more than 2,000 women, those with high triglycerides and low HDL had a significant risk of developing breast cancer (Berrino et al., 2014).

In a study of postmenopausal African American women, the presence of symptoms of metabolic syndrome was associated with the development of breast cancer (Bosco, Palmer, Boggs, Hatch, & Rosenberg, 2012); however, the authors cautioned that it is not individual factors but the combination of central obesity, type 2 diabetes, hypertension, and high cholesterol that increases the risk of breast cancer for this population. In another example, increased WHR in Asian women was found to be associated with an increased risk of premenopausal breast cancer. Caucasian and African American women were not found to be at an increased risk based on WHR (Amadou et al., 2013). Kwan et al. (2014) suggested that BMI may be a better indicator of survival in obese Caucasian and Latina women, while central adiposity may be a better indicator for Asian and African American women.

Short-term weight gain, which is defined as gaining 15 lb (6.8 kg) or more in four years, increases the risk of breast cancer in premenopausal women of a healthy weight by 38%. This is compared to postmenopausal women of a healthy weight, where the risk is increased by 10% (Rosner et al., 2015).

In a study of women attending a breast center, almost 60% of patients were overweight or obese (Kim et al., 2014). Sixty-four percent of the overweight or obese women had been diagnosed with breast cancer, and 65% were at high risk (Gail risk score ≥ 1.66%, *BRCA*-mutation positive, significant family history of breast cancer, abnormal proliferative lesion on breast biopsy) compared to women of normal weight, where 35.8% had breast cancer and 35% were at high risk.

Inflammation may be one factor contributing to the development of breast cancer. The presence of C-reactive protein, an inflammatory marker, was found to raise the risk of breast cancer in postmenopausal women (Gunter et al., 2015). Obesity is also strongly associated with insulin resistance, chronic inflammation, and secretion of adipokines, all of which are associated with tumor progression (Fuentes-Mattei et al., 2014; van Kruijsdijk, van der Wall, & Visseren, 2009).

A sedentary lifestyle also has been suggested as a causative factor in postmenopausal women (Wiseman, Lynch, Cameron, & Dunstan, 2014). Women with breast cancer also have a poorer prognosis when they are not physically active, with one review suggesting a 30% increased risk of mortality (Patterson, Cadmus, Emond, & Pierce, 2010). Obesity in women with breast cancer has been shown to result in lower quality of life and an increased risk of cardiovascular disease, which further contributes to impaired physical functioning and quality of life (Elme et al., 2013).

Obesity has also been suggested to play a role in the development of triple-negative breast cancer with poorer disease markers, including larger tumors and higher tumor grade (Mowad et al., 2013). However, obesity was not seen to affect survival in women with these kinds of tumors (Tait et al., 2014). It has also been suggested that obesity results in less effective suppression of estrogen in the tissues of women treated with aromatase inhibitors; however, the evidence to date is not well established. Some studies have shown no effect of obesity on anastrozole metabolism (Hubalek et al., 2014; Lonning, Haynes, & Dowsett, 2014), while one small study suggested that aromatase inhibitors are less effective when used in obese women (Pfeiler et al., 2013). This should be interpreted with caution until larger studies are conducted.

Prostate Cancer

Although the relationship between obesity and prostate cancer has not clearly been explained to date, it appears that the two are related—more so in poor outcomes for obese men with prostate cancer. However, a meta-analysis of more than two million men in 25 studies concluded that obesity appears to decrease localized disease and increase the risk for advanced disease (Discacciati, Orsini, & Wolk, 2012). For localized cancer, for every 5 kg/m^2 increase in BMI, the relative risk was 0.94 (95% confidence interval [CI] [0.91, 0.97]). For advanced cancer, however, the relative risk for every 5 kg/m^2 increase in BMI was 1.09 (95% CI [1.02, 1.16]). These findings were confirmed by a study of 6,729 men that showed a decreased risk of low-grade cancer and an increased risk of aggressive cancer (Vidal et al., 2014). An earlier meta-analysis of observational studies reported no increased risk (Renehan, Tyson, Egger, Heller, & Zwahlen, 2008).

In their 2012 meta-analysis, Discacciati et al. suggested that although the reasons for this dual relationship are not clear, testosterone may be implicated. This concept was studied by a group from Germany. Although obesity was associated with the development of aggressive prostate cancer, the authors found that testosterone was not a causative factor. Rather, low levels of testosterone were found in obese men (Jentzmik et al., 2014).

Gynecologic Cancer

It is well established that obesity plays a role in the development of gynecologic cancers, especially uterine/endometrial cancer. Obesity is associated with younger age at diagnosis (Nevadunsky et al., 2014), and being overweight at age 20 is associated with an almost twofold increased risk (hazard ratio [HR] 1.83, 95% CI [1.4, 2.37]) (Dougan et al., 2015). The presence of metabolic syndrome is associated with an increased risk of endometrial cancer (odds ratio [OR] 1.39, 95% CI [1.31, 1.47]) and overweight and obesity itself with 95% increased risk (OR 1.95, 95% CI [1.9, 2.11]) (Trabert et al., 2015). Being overweight at age 18 and weight gain during adulthood also have been associated with an increased risk of developing endometrial cancer in women who have not used hormone therapy in their postmenopausal years (Stevens et al., 2014). In women younger than age 49, excess weight and presumed excess estrogen were seen as contributing factors in the development of endometrial cancer in a population of 719 women, 57.5% of whom were obese (Burleigh, Talhouk, Gilks, & McAlpine, 2015).

Being overweight or mildly obese confers risk for cervical cancer (OR 1.25, 95% CI [0.79, 2.0]; and OR 1.70, 95% CI [1.10, 2.63], respectively) (Lee, So, Piyathilake, & Kim, 2013). The risk for ovarian cancer is associated with obesity (HR 2.90, 95% CI [1.30, 6.46]) (Wu et al., 2014). African American women who are overweight or obese often have an increased risk of ovarian cancer (Schildkraut et al., 2014).

Colorectal Cancer

The association between colorectal cancer and overweight and obesity is well known. In a meta-analysis of 56 studies including more than 93,000 individuals with colorectal cancer (Ning, Wang, & Giovannucci, 2010), colorectal cancer risk was increased by 19% in those with a BMI of 25–27.4 kg/m^2 and by 24% in those with a BMI of 27.5–29.9 kg/m^2. For obese individuals (BMI ≥ 30 kg/m^2), the risk of developing colorectal cancer was 41% higher as compared to normal-weight individuals. Weight loss or prevention of weight gain is regarded as one way of preventing the occurrence of colorectal cancer (Chan et al., 2010). Obesity also is associated with an increased risk of more advanced cancer on diagnosis (OR 3.83, 95% CI [1.94, 7.55]) (Stein et al., 2010). Overweight African American men are at higher risk of developing colorectal cancer (Ashktorab et al., 2014). Weight gain over time is also associated with an increased risk of colorectal cancer. In a large prospective study of 201,696 participants, weight gain between the ages of 20 and 50 was associated with a 60% increased risk of colon cancer (95% CI [1.2, 2.09]) (Aleksandrova et al., 2013). It has also been noted that overweight and obese individuals do not recognize that their weight places them at increased risk (Fagan, Sifri, Wender, Schumacher, & Reed, 2012), and so they may not participate in the recommended screening that could identify precancerous changes and prevent the development of more advanced disease.

Other Cancers

Although the preponderance of evidence linking overweight and obesity and cancer lies in breast, prostate, gynecologic, and colorectal cancers, associations have been found for other cancers. Kidney cancer is associated with obesity, with younger patients being diagnosed who are overweight or obese (McGuire & Fitzpatric, 2011). In a summary analysis of 14 studies, the relative risk (RR) of being diagnosed with renal cancer was 1.07 for each increased unit of BMI (95% CI [1.05, 1.09]) (Bergström et al., 2001). Obesity and hypertension were found to be associated with renal cancer in a very large sample of men and women (N = 510,114), although the etiology is not known (Sanfilippo et al., 2014). As with other cancers, the general public has a low level of knowledge related to the association of overweight and obesity and renal cancer (Parker, Arnold, Diehl, Hassan, & Thiel, 2014).

The risk of thyroid cancer is associated with obesity (RR 1.33, 95% CI [1.24, 1.42]); particular subtypes of thyroid cancer include papillary, follicular, and anaplastic (Ma et al., 2015). In another study (Xu et al., 2014), the risk of papillary thyroid cancer was found to be related to overweight (OR 1.72, 95% CI [1.48, 2.0]) and obesity (OR 4.17, 95% CI [3.41, 5.10]).

Abdominal obesity, as measured by waist circumference, was found to be a risk factor for esophageal adenocarcinoma (Steffen et al., 2015).

Risk of Recurrence and Mortality

Obesity and overweight have also been associated with poorer outcomes, including recurrence and mortality. For example, obesity was found to be associated with an increased risk of death in African Americans with pancreatic cancer (OR 1.25, 95%

CI [0.99, 1.57]) and a BMI of 30–34.9 kg/m^2 (Bethea et al., 2014). Obesity can also be linked to various other cancers, including the following.

Breast Cancer

Weight gain after the diagnosis of breast cancer is common and is influenced by many factors, including age, menopausal status, ethnicity, smoking status, and endocrine therapies (Sedjo et al., 2014). A number of recent studies highlight the increased risk of poor prognosis in women with breast cancer who are overweight or obese.

Higher BMI in asymptomatic women with screen-detected breast cancer is associated with lower disease-free and overall survival (Crispo et al., 2015). Moderate to severe obesity is associated with recurrence of disease independent of age, even in women on adjuvant endocrine therapy (Robinson, Bell, & Davis, 2014), and the effects of endocrine therapy in preventing recurrence appear to be lost more rapidly in obese women (Ewertz et al., 2011). The class of endocrine therapy (aromatase inhibitor versus selective estrogen receptor modulator [SERM]) may be important for overall survival. One study showed letrozole to be of greater benefit for obese women (Ewertz et al., 2012); however, it is suggested that BMI should not be used as a rationale for choosing an aromatase inhibitor over a SERM to prevent recurrence (Goodwin, 2013).

In another study, overweight and obese women had an almost twofold increased risk of poor prognosis compared to normal-weight women (Arce-Salinas et al., 2014). In another study, obese women had more extensive tumors and a 32% increased risk of recurrence (Majed et al., 2008). Another large study reported that only morbidly obese women (and underweight women) had an increased risk for mortality, while women who were classified as overweight did not experience excess risk (Kwan et al., 2012). Yet another study showed that obesity was associated with a decrease in recurrence-free, overall, and breast cancer–specific survival in women with ER-positive disease. The presence of diabetes had a negative effect on recurrence-free and overall survival; given the association between obesity and diabetes, control of both was seen to be important in improving survival (Jiralerspong et al., 2013). An increased risk of recurrence and death persists in obese women for at least 10 years after diagnosis (Kamineni et al., 2013). To date, no association has been established between overweight and obesity and poorer prognosis in triple-negative breast cancer (Ademuyiwa et al., 2011; Dawood et al., 2012).

Weight gain of 5% or greater after diagnosis is associated with an increased risk of all-cause mortality (HR 1.12, 95% CI [1.03, 1.22]). Although those with a weight gain of 5%–10% show no significant increase in mortality, women who experience weight gain of 10% or greater have a 23% risk of mortality (HR 1.23, 95% CI [1.09, 1.39]) (Playdon et al., 2015).

Prostate Cancer

Obesity at the time of diagnosis of prostate cancer is associated with higher mortality, including prostate-specific mortality (HR 1.44, 95% CI [1.09, 1.90]) and overall mortality (HR 1.33, 95% CI [1.09, 1.63]) (Cantarutti et al., 2015). Another study showed that obese men have a 50% increased risk of dying from prostate cancer when compared to normal-weight men (OR 1.50, 95% CI [1.03, 2.19]). For men with high-risk prostate cancer (Gleason score of 8 or higher), the risk of dying is even higher (OR 2.37, 95% CI [1.11, 5.09]) (Haque et al., 2014).

Studies in men being treated validate the poor outcomes for obese men. For men treated with radiation therapy, obesity increases the risk of recurrence, distant metastases, and prostate-specific mortality (Wang et al., 2015). Obesity is a factor in the risk of recurrence for men after radical prostatectomy; 20-year actuarial recurrence-free survival in obese men was much lower than in healthy weight men at 51% compared to 76% ($p < 0.001$) (Chalfin et al., 2014). For men with low-risk prostate cancer considering active surveillance as a treatment modality, obesity increased the risk of eventual upgrading and upstaging of the cancer and seminal vesicle invasion by about 22% (de Cobelli et al., 2015). An earlier study also found an increased risk for disease progression in men on active surveillance (Bhindi et al., 2014). In a meta-analysis of more than one million men with prostate cancer, a 5 kg/m^2 increase in BMI was associated with a 15% increased risk of dying from prostate cancer (Cao & Ma, 2011). Given how common prostate cancer is and the large number of men who are obese in the general population, this results in a significant number of men who will die from prostate cancer in part because of the added risk of their weight.

In addition to an increased risk of mortality, obesity increases the incidence of intraoperative complications and postoperative urinary incontinence, affecting quality of life (Gacci et al., 2014; Wolin, Luly, Sutcliffe, Andriole, & Kibel, 2010).

Gynecologic Cancer

Being morbidly obese predisposes women to poorer outcomes after treatment for all gynecologic cancers, including endometrial cancer, where quality of life is decreased and the risk of surgical complications is higher (Bouwman et al., 2015; Mahdi, Jernigan, Aljebori, Lockhart, & Moslemi-Kebria, 2015; Smits, Lopes, Das, Bekkers, & Galaal, 2014). A systematic review reported that obese women with endometrial cancer have higher all-cause mortality after treatment (Arem & Irwin, 2013). Obesity has been shown to increase morbidity in women treated for cervical cancer; these women are at increased risk for weight gain after treatment (Schlumbrecht, Sun, Huang, Zandstra, & Bodurka, 2014). Morbid obesity also is an independent risk factor for dying from cervical cancer (Frumovitz et al., 2014). In women treated for ovarian cancer, increased BMI has been shown to result in poorer physical and emotional quality of life (Smits, Lopes, Das, Bekkers, & Galaal, 2015). Morbidly obese women with ovarian cancer are at risk for surgical complications within 30 days and increased risk of death 90 days after surgery to debulk the tumor (Kumar, Bakkum-Gamez, Weaver, McGree, & Cliby, 2014). For women with recurrent ovarian cancer, obesity is associated with poorer overall survival (Tran, Cohen, & Li, 2015).

Colorectal Cancer

Obesity is a risk factor for colorectal cancer recurrence (Scarpa et al., 2014) as well as the development of a secondary cancer. For every five-unit change in BMI, the risk of developing another cancer, usually one associated with obesity, increases 12% (Gibson et al., 2014). Obese women who are postmenopausal are at double the risk of dying from colorectal cancer than normal-weight women (HR 2.1, 95% CI [1.1, 3.8]) (Doria-Rose, Newcomb, Morimoto, Hampton, & Trentham-Dietz, 2006). Elevated BMI at the time of diagnosis, but not after treatment, has been shown to increase the risk of dying from colorectal cancer (RR 1.35, 95% CI [1.01, 1.80]) and all-cause mortality (RR 1.30, 95% CI [1.06, 1.58]) (Campbell et al., 2012). This also was shown in another study, where the risk of women dying from colorectal cancer was almost twice as high in overweight women (HR 1.5, 95% CI [1.04, 2.18]) (Boyle, Fritschi, Platell, & Heyworth, 2013).

Conclusion

The contemporary studies cited in this chapter highlight the strong evidence for both the development of and poor outcomes for specific cancers, many of which are common. Because of this, large numbers of affected individuals have modifiable risk factors that could have prevented the occurrence of the cancer or reduced the risk of unfavorable outcomes. It is highly likely that as the evidence continues to grow, other cancers will be found to be associated with overweight and obesity, and healthcare providers will have stronger evidence to promote weight loss and prevention of weight gain as primary prevention for these additional cancers.

References

Ademuyiwa, F.O., Groman, A., O'Connor, T., Ambrosone, C., Watroba, N., & Edge, S.B. (2011). Impact of body mass index on clinical outcomes in triple-negative breast cancer. *Cancer, 117,* 4132–4140. doi:10.1002/cncr.26019

Aleksandrova, K., Pischon, T., Buijsse, B., May, A.M., Peeters, P.H., Bueno-de-Mesquita, H.B., … Boeing, H. (2013). Adult weight change and risk of colorectal cancer in the European prospective investigation into cancer and nutrition. *European Journal of Cancer, 49,* 3526–3536. doi:10.1016/j.ejca.2013.06.021

Amadou, A., Ferrari, P., Muwonge, R., Moskal, A., Biessy, C., Romieu, I., & Hainaut, P. (2013). Overweight, obesity and risk of premenopausal breast cancer according to ethnicity: A systematic review and dose-response meta-analysis. *Obesity Reviews, 14,* 665–678. doi:10.1111/obr.12028

Arce-Salinas, C., Aguilar-Ponce, J.L., Villarreal-Garza, C., Lara-Medina, F.U., Olvera-Caraza, D., Alvarado Miranda, A., … Mohar, A. (2014). Overweight and obesity as poor prognostic factors in locally advanced breast cancer patients. *Breast Cancer Research and Treatment, 146,* 183–188. doi:10.1007/s10549-014-2977-8

Arem, H., & Irwin, M.L. (2013). Obesity and endometrial cancer survival: A systematic review. *International Journal of Obesity, 37,* 634–639. doi:10.1038/ijo.2012.94

Ashktorab, H., Paydar, M., Yazdi, S., Namin, H.H., Sanderson, A., Begum, R., … Nouraie, M. (2014). BMI and the risk of colorectal adenoma in African Americans. *Obesity, 22,* 1387–1391. doi:10.1002/oby.20702

Bandera, E.V., Chandran, U., Hong, C.C., Troester, M.A., Bethea, T.N., Adams-Campbell, L.L., … Rosenberg, L. (2015). Obesity, body fat distribution, and risk of breast cancer subtypes in African American women participating in the AMBER Consortium. *Breast Cancer Research and Treatment, 150,* 655–666. doi:10.1007/s10549-015-3353-z

Bergström, A., Hsieh, C.C., Lindblad, P., Lu, C.M., Cook, N.R., & Wolk, A. (2001). Obesity and renal cell cancer—A quantitative review. *British Journal of Cancer, 85,* 984–990. doi:10.1054/bjoc.2001.2040

Berrino, F., Villarini, A., Traina, A., Bonanni, B., Panico, S., Mano, M.P., … Pasanisi, P. (2014). Metabolic syndrome and breast cancer prognosis. *Breast Cancer Research and Treatment, 147,* 159–165. doi:10.1007/s10549-014-3076-6

Bethea, T.N., Kitahara, C.M., Sonderman, J., Patel, A.V., Harvey, C., Knutsen, S.F., … Kolonel, L.N. (2014). A pooled analysis of body mass index and pancreatic cancer mortality in African Americans. *Cancer Epidemiology, Biomarkers and Prevention, 23,* 2119–2125. doi:10.1158/1055-9965.EPI-14-0422

Bhindi, B., Kulkarni, G.S., Finelli, A., Alibhai, S.M.H., Hamilton, R.J., Toi, A., … Fleshner, N.E. (2014). Obesity is associated with risk of progression for low-risk prostate cancers managed expectantly. *European Urology, 66,* 841–848. doi:10.1016/j.eururo.2014.06.005

Bosco, J.L.F., Palmer, J.R., Boggs, D.A., Hatch, E.E., & Rosenberg, L. (2012). Cardiometabolic factors and breast cancer risk in U.S. black women. *Breast Cancer Research and Treatment, 134,* 1247–1256. doi:10.1007/s10549-012-2131-4

Bouwman, F., Smits, A., Lopes, A., Das, N., Pollard, A., Massuger, L., … Galaal, K. (2015). The impact of BMI on surgical complications and outcomes in endometrial cancer surgery—An institutional study and systematic review of the literature. *Gynecologic Oncology, 139,* 369–376. doi:10.1016/j.ygyno.2015.09.020

Boyle, T., Fritschi, L., Platell, C., & Heyworth, J. (2013). Lifestyle factors associated with survival after colorectal cancer diagnosis. *British Journal of Cancer, 109,* 814–822. doi:10.1038/bjc.2013.310

Burleigh, A., Talhouk, A., Gilks, C.B., & McAlpine, J.N. (2015). Clinical and pathological characterization of endometrial cancer in young women: Identification of a cohort without classical risk factors. *Gynecologic Oncology, 138,* 141–146. doi:10.1016/j.ygyno.2015.02.028

Campbell, P.T., Newton, C.C., Dehal, A.N., Jacobs, E.J., Patel, A.V., & Gapstur, S.M. (2012). Impact of body mass index on survival after colorectal cancer diagnosis: The Cancer Prevention Study-II Nutrition Cohort. *Journal of Clinical Oncology, 30,* 42–52. doi:10.1200/JCO.2011.38.0287

Cantarutti, A., Bonn, S.E., Adami, H.O., Grönberg, H., Bellocco, R., & Bälter, K. (2015). Body mass index and mortality in men with prostate cancer. *Prostate, 75,* 1129–1136. doi:10.1002/pros.23001

Cao, Y., & Ma, J. (2011). Body mass index, prostate cancer–specific mortality, and biochemical recurrence: A systematic review and meta-analysis. *Cancer Prevention Research, 4,* 486–501. doi:10.1158/1940-6207.CAPR-10-0229

Chalfin, H.J., Lee, S.B., Jeong, B.C., Freedland, S.J., Alai, H., Feng, Z., … Han, M. (2014). Obesity and long-term survival after radical prostatectomy. *Journal of Urology, 192,* 1100–1104. doi:10.1016/j.juro.2014.04.086

Chan, D.S., & Norat, T. (2015). Obesity and breast cancer: Not only a risk factor of the disease. *Current Treatment Options in Oncology, 16*(5), 22. doi:10.1007/s11864-015-0341-9

Chan, K.K., Dassanayake, B., Deen, R., Wickramarachchi, R.E., Kumarage, S.K., Samita, S., & Deen, K.I. (2010). Young patients with colorectal cancer have poor survival in the first twenty months after operation and predictable survival in the medium and long-term: Analysis of survival and prognostic markers. *World Journal of Surgical Oncology, 8,* 82. doi:10.1186/1477-7819-8-82

Chlebowski, R.T., Aiello, E., & McTiernan, A. (2002). Weight loss in breast cancer patient management. *Journal of Clinical Oncology, 20,* 1128–1143. doi:10.1200/JCO.20.4.1128

Cleary, M.P., & Grossman, M.E. (2009). Minireview: Obesity and breast cancer: The estrogen connection. *Endocrinology, 150,* 2537–2542. doi:10.1210/en.2009-0070

Copson, E.R., Cutress, R.I., Maishman, T., Eccles, B.K., Gerty, S., Stanton, L., ... Eccles, D.M. (2015). Obesity and the outcome of young breast cancer patients in the UK: The POSH study. *Annals of Oncology, 26,* 101–112. doi:10.1093/annonc/mdu509

Crispo, A., Grimaldi, M., D'Aiuto, M., Rinaldo, M., Capasso, I., Amore, A., ... Montella, M. (2015). BMI and breast cancer prognosis benefit: Mammography screening reveals differences between normal weight and overweight women. *Breast, 24,* 86–89. doi:10.1016/j.breast.2014.11.005

Dawood, S., Lei, X., Litton, J.K., Buchholz, T.A., Hortobagyi, G.N., & Gonzalez-Angulo, A.M. (2012). Impact of body mass index on survival outcome among women with early stage triple-negative breast cancer. *Clinical Breast Cancer, 12,* 364–372. doi:10.1016/j.clbc.2012.07.013

de Cobelli, O., Terracciano, D., Tagliabue, E., Raimondi, S., Galasso, G., Cioffi, A., ... Ferro, M. (2015). Body mass index was associated with upstaging and upgrading in patients with low-risk prostate cancer who met the inclusion criteria for active surveillance. *Urologic Oncology, 33,* 201.e1–201.e8. doi:10.1016/j.urolonc.2015.02.004

Discacciati, A., Orsini, N., & Wolk, A. (2012). Body mass index and incidence of localized and advanced prostate cancer—A dose–response meta-analysis of prospective studies. *Annals of Oncology, 23,* 1665–1671. doi:10.1093/annonc/mdr603

Doria-Rose, V.P., Newcomb, P.A., Morimoto, L.M., Hampton, J.M., & Trentham-Dietz, A. (2006). Body mass index and the risk of death following the diagnosis of colorectal cancer in postmenopausal women (United States). *Cancer Causes and Control, 17,* 63–70. doi:10.1007/s10552-005-0360-0

Dougan, M.M., Hankinson, S.E., Vivo, I.D., Tworoger, S.S., Glynn, R.J., & Michels, K.B. (2015). Prospective study of body size throughout the life-course and the incidence of endometrial cancer among premenopausal and postmenopausal women. *International Journal of Cancer, 137,* 625–637. doi:10.1002/ijc.29427

Druesne-Pecollo, N., Touvier, M., Barrandon, E., Chan, D.S., Norat, T., Zelek, L., ... Latino-Martel, P. (2012). Excess body weight and second primary cancer risk after breast cancer: A systematic review and meta-analysis of prospective studies. *Breast Cancer Research and Treatment, 135,* 647–654. doi:10.1007/s10549-012-2187-1

Elme, A., Utriainen, M., Kellokumpu-Lehtinen, P., Palva, T., Luoto, R., Nikander, R., ... Saarto, T. (2013). Obesity and physical inactivity are related to impaired physical health of breast cancer survivors. *Anticancer Research, 33,* 1595–1602.

Ewertz, M., Gray, K.P., Regan, M.M., Ejlertsen, B., Price, K.N., Thürlimann, B., ... Mouridsen, H.T. (2012). Obesity and risk of recurrence or death after adjuvant endocrine therapy with letrozole or tamoxifen in the Breast International Group 1-98 trial. *Journal of Clinical Oncology, 30,* 3967–3975. doi:10.1200/JCO.2011.40.8666

Ewertz, M., Jensen, M.B., Gunnarsdóttir, K.Á., Højris, I., Jakobsen, E.H., Nielsen, D., ... Cold, S. (2011). Effect of obesity on prognosis after early-stage breast cancer. *Journal of Clinical Oncology, 29,* 25–31. doi:10.1200/JCO.2010.29.7614

Fagan, H.B., Sifri, R., Wender, R., Schumacher, E., & Reed, J.F., III. (2012). Weight status and perception of colorectal cancer risk. *Journal of the American Board of Family Medicine, 25,* 792–797. doi:10.3122/jabfm.2012.06.120017

Fontanella, C., Lederer, B., Gade, S., Vanoppen, M., Blohmer, J.U., Costa, S.D., ... Loibl, S. (2015). Impact of body mass index on neoadjuvant treatment outcome: A pooled analysis of eight prospective neoadjuvant breast cancer trials. *Breast Cancer Research and Treatment, 150,* 127–139. doi:10.1007/s10549-015-3287-5

Frumovitz, M., Jhingran, A., Soliman, P.T., Klopp, A.H., Schmeler, K.M., & Eifel, P.J. (2014). Morbid obesity as an independent risk factor for disease-specific mortality in women with cervical cancer. *Obstetrics and Gynecology, 124,* 1098–1104. doi:10.1097/AOG.0000000000000558

Fuentes-Mattei, E., Velazquez-Torres, G., Phan, L., Zhang, F., Chou, P.-C., Shin, J.-H., ... Yeung, S.-C. (2014). Effects of obesity on transcriptomic changes and cancer hallmarks in estrogen receptor-positive breast cancer. *Journal of the National Cancer Institute, 106.* doi:10.1093/jnci/dju158

Gacci, M., Sebastianelli, A., Salvi, M., De Nunzio, C., Schiavina, R., Simonato, A., ... Carmignani, G. (2014). Role of abdominal obesity for functional outcomes and complications in men treated with radical prostatectomy for prostate cancer: Results of the Multicenter Italian Report on Radical Prostatectomy (MIRROR) study. *Scandinavian Journal of Urology, 48,* 138–145. doi:10.3109/21681805.2013.803151

Gibson, T.M., Park, Y., Robien, K., Shiels, M.S., Black, A., Sampson, J.N., ... Morton, L.M. (2014). Body mass index and risk of second obesity-associated cancers after colorectal cancer: A pooled analysis of prospective cohort studies. *Journal of Clinical Oncology, 32,* 4004–4011. doi:10.1200/JCO.2014.56.8444

Goodwin, P.J. (2013). Obesity and endocrine therapy: Host factors and breast cancer outcome. *Breast, 22*(Suppl. 2), S44–S47. doi:10.1016/j.breast.2013.07.008

Gunter, M.J., Wang, T., Cushman, M., Xue, X., Wassertheil-Smoller, S., Strickler, H.D., ... Ho, G.Y. (2015). Circulating adipokines and inflammatory markers and postmenopausal breast cancer risk. *Journal of the National Cancer Institute, 107.* doi:10.1093/jnci/djv169

Haque, R., Van Den Eeden, S.K., Wallner, L.P., Richert-Boe, K., Kallakury, B., Wang, R., & Weinmann, S. (2014). Association of body mass index and prostate cancer mortality. *Obesity Research and Clinical Practice, 8,* e374–e381. doi:10.1016/j.orcp.2013.06.002

Heo, M., Kabat, G.C., Strickler, H.D., Lin, J., Hou, L., Stefanick, M.L., ... Rohan, T.E. (2015). Optimal cutoffs of obesity measures in relation to cancer risk in postmenopausal women in the Women's Health Initiative Study. *Journal of Women's Health, 24,* 218–227. doi:10.1089/jwh.2014.4977

Hubalek, M., Oberguggenberger, A., Beer, B., Meraner, V., Sztankay, M., Oberacher, H., ... Sperner-Unterweger, B. (2014). Does obesity interfere with anastrozole treatment? Positive association between body mass index and anastrozole plasma levels. *Clinical Breast Cancer, 14,* 291–296. doi:10.1016/j.clbc.2013.12.008

Jentzmik, F., Schnoeller, T.J., Cronauer, M.V., Steinestel, J., Steffens, S., Zengerling, F., ... Schrader, A.J. (2014). Corpulence is the crucial factor: Association of testosterone and/or obesity with prostate cancer stage. *International Journal of Urology, 21,* 980–986. doi:10.1111/iju.12494

Jiralerspong, S., Kim, E.S., Dong, W., Feng, L., Hortobagyi, G.N., & Giordano, S.H. (2013). Obesity, diabetes, and survival outcomes in a large cohort of early-stage breast cancer patients. *Annals of Oncology, 24,* 2506–2514. doi:10.1093/annonc/mdt224

Kamineni, A., Anderson, M.L., White, E., Taplin, S.H., Porter, P., Ballard-Barbash, R., ... Buist, D.S. (2013). Body mass index, tumor characteristics, and prognosis following diagnosis of early-stage breast cancer in a mammographically screened population. *Cancer Causes and Control, 24,* 305–312. doi:10.1007/s10552-012-0115-7

Kim, A., Scharf, K., Senthil, M., Solomon, N., Garberoglio, C., & Lum, S.S. (2014). The prevalence of overweight and obesity in a breast clinic population: Consideration for weight loss as a therapeutic intervention. *Surgery for Obesity and Related Diseases, 10,* 348–353. doi:10.1016/j.soard.2013.07.019

Kumar, A., Bakkum-Gamez, J.N., Weaver, A.L., McGree, M.E., & Cliby, W.A. (2014). Impact of obesity on surgical and oncologic outcomes in ovarian cancer. *Gynecologic Oncology, 135,* 19–24. doi:10.1016/j.ygyno.2014.07.103

Kwan, M.L., Chen, W.Y., Kroenke, C.H., Weltzien, E.K., Beasley, J.M., Nechuta, S.J., ... Caan, B.J. (2012). Pre-diagnosis body mass index and survival after breast cancer in the after breast cancer pooling project. *Breast Cancer Research and Treatment, 132,* 729–739. doi:10.1007/s10549-011-1914-3

Kwan, M.L., John, E.M., Caan, B.J., Lee, V.S., Bernstein, L., Cheng, I., ... Wu, A.H. (2014). Obesity and mortality after breast cancer by race/ethnicity: The California Breast Cancer Survivorship Consortium. *American Journal of Epidemiology, 179,* 95–111. doi:10.1093/aje/kwt233

Lee, J.K., So, K.A., Piyathilake, C.J., & Kim, M.K. (2013). Mild obesity, physical activity, calorie intake, and the risks of cervical intraepithelial neoplasia and cervical cancer. *PLOS ONE, 8,* e66555. doi:10.1371/journal.pone.0066555

Lonning, P.E., Haynes, B.P., & Dowsett, M. (2014). Relationship of body mass index with aromatisation and plasma and tissue oestrogen levels in postmenopausal breast cancer patients treated with aromatase inhibitors. *European Journal of Cancer, 50,* 1055–1064. doi:10.1016/j.ejca.2014.01.007

Ma, J., Huang, M., Wang, L., Ye, W., Tong, Y., & Wang, H. (2015). Obesity and risk of thyroid cancer: Evidence from a meta-analysis of 21 observational studies. *Medical Science Monitor, 21,* 283–291. doi:10.12659/MSM.892035

Mahdi, H., Jernigan, A.M., Aljebori, Q., Lockhart, D., & Moslemi-Kebria, M. (2015). The impact of obesity on the 30-day morbidity and mortality after surgery for endometrial cancer. *Journal of Minimally Invasive Gynecology, 22,* 94–102. doi:10.1016/j.jmig.2014.07.014

Majed, B., Moreau, T., Senouci, K., Salmon, R.J., Fourquet, A., & Asselain, B. (2008). Is obesity an independent prognosis factor in woman breast cancer? *Breast Cancer Research and Treatment, 111,* 329–342. doi:10.1007/s10549-007-9785-3

McGuire, B.B., & Fitzpatric, J.M. (2011). BMI and the risk of renal cell carcinoma. *Current Opinion in Urology, 21,* 356–361. doi:10.1097/MOU.0b013e32834962d5

Montazeri, A. (2008). Health-related quality of life in breast cancer patients: A bibliographic review of the literature from 1974 to 2007. *Journal of Experimental and Clinical Cancer Research, 27,* 1–31. doi:10.1186/1756-9966-27-32

Mowad, R., Chu, Q.D., Li, B.D., Burton, G.V., Ampil, F.L., & Kim, R.H. (2013). Does obesity have an effect on outcomes in triple-negative breast cancer? *Journal of Surgical Research, 184,* 253–259. doi:10.1016/j.jss.2013.05.037

Nevadunsky, N.S., Van Arsdale, A., Strickler, H.D., Moadel, A., Kaur, G., Levitt, J., ... Einstein, M.H. (2014). Obesity and age at diagnosis of endometrial cancer. *Obstetrics and Gynecology, 124,* 300–306. doi:10.1097/AOG.0000000000000381

Ning, Y., Wang, L., & Giovannucci, E.L. (2010). A quantitative analysis of body mass index and colorectal cancer: Findings from 56 observational studies. *Obesity Reviews, 11,* 19–30. doi:10.1111/j.1467-789X.2009.00613.x

Niraula, S., Ocana, A., Ennis, M., & Goodwin, P.J. (2012). Body size and breast cancer prognosis in relation to hormone receptor and menopausal status: A meta-analysis. *Breast Cancer Research and Treatment, 134,* 769–781. doi:10.1007/s10549-012-2073-x

Parker, A.S., Arnold, M.L., Diehl, N.D., Hassan, L., & Thiel, D.D. (2014). Evaluation of awareness of risk factors for kidney cancer among patients presenting to a urology clinic. *Scandinavian Journal of Urology, 48,* 239–244. doi:10.3109/21681805.2013.863803

Patterson, R.E., Cadmus, L.A., Emond, J.A., & Pierce, J.P. (2010). Physical activity, diet, adiposity and female breast cancer prognosis: A review of the epidemiologic literature. *Maturitas, 66,* 5–15. doi:10.1016/j.maturitas.2010.01.004

Pfeiler, G., Königsberg, R., Hadji, P., Fitzal, F., Maroske, M., Dressel-Ban, G., ... Dubsky, P. (2013). Impact of body mass index on estradiol depletion by aromatase inhibitors in postmenopausal women with early breast cancer. *British Journal of Cancer, 109,* 1522–1527. doi:10.1038/bjc.2013.499

Playdon, M.C., Bracken, M.B., Sanft, T.B., Ligibel, J.A., Harrigan, M., & Irwin, M.L. (2015). Weight gain after breast cancer diagnosis and all-cause mortality: Systematic review and meta-analysis. *Journal of the National Cancer Institute, 107,* djv275. doi:10.1093/jnci/djv275

Protani, M., Coory, M., & Martin, J.H. (2010). Effect of obesity on survival of women with breast cancer: Systematic review and meta-analysis. *Breast Cancer Research and Treatment, 123,* 627–635. doi:10.1007/s10549-010-0990-0

Renehan, A.G., Tyson, M., Egger, M., Heller, R.F., & Zwahlen, M. (2008). Body-mass index and incidence of cancer: A systematic review and meta-analysis of prospective observational studies. *Lancet, 371,* 569–578. doi:10.1016/S0140-6736(08)60269-X

Robinson, P.J., Bell, R.J., & Davis, S.R. (2014). Obesity is associated with a poorer prognosis in women with hormone receptor positive breast cancer. *Maturitas, 79,* 279–286. doi:10.1016/j.maturitas.2014.07.004

Rosner, B., Eliassen, A.H., Toriola, A.T., Hankinson, S.E., Willett, W.C., Natarajan, L., & Colditz, G.A. (2015). Short-term weight gain and breast cancer risk by hormone receptor classification among pre- and postmenopausal women. *Breast Cancer Research and Treatment, 150,* 643–653. doi:10.1007/s10549-015-3344-0

Sanfilippo, K.M., McTigue, K.M., Fidler, C.J., Neaton, J.D., Chang, Y., Fried, L.F., ... Kuller, L.H. (2014). Hypertension and obesity and the risk of kidney cancer in 2 large cohorts of US men and women. *Hypertension, 63,* 934–941. doi:10.1161/hypertensionaha.113.02953

Scarpa, M., Ruffolo, C., Erroi, F., Fiorot, A., Basato, S., Pozza, A., ... Castoro, C. (2014). Obesity is a risk factor for multifocal disease and recurrence after colorectal cancer surgery: A case-control study. *Anticancer Research, 34,* 5735–5741.

Schildkraut, J.M., Alberg, A.J., Bandera, E.V., Barnholtz-Sloan, J., Bondy, M., Cote, M.L., … Moorman, P.G. (2014). A multi-center population-based case-control study of ovarian cancer in African-American women: The African American Cancer Epidemiology Study (AACES). *BMC Cancer, 14,* 688. doi:10.1186/1471-2407-14-688

Schlumbrecht, M.P., Sun, C.C., Huang, M.S., Zandstra, F., & Bodurka, D.C. (2014). Lifestyle modification in cervical cancer survivors: An ongoing need. *International Journal of Gynecologic Cancer, 24,* 570–575. doi:10.1097/IGC.0000000000000081

Sedjo, R.L., Byers, T., Ganz, P.A., Colditz, G.A., Demark-Wahnefried, W., Wolin, K.Y., … Rock, C.L. (2014). Weight gain prior to entry into a weight-loss intervention study among overweight and obese breast cancer survivors. *Journal of Cancer Survivorship, 8,* 410–418. doi:10.1007/s11764-014-0351-9

Smits, A., Lopes, A., Das, N., Bekkers, R., & Galaal, K. (2014). The impact of BMI on quality of life in obese endometrial cancer survivors: Does size matter? *Gynecologic Oncology, 132,* 137–141. doi:10.1016/j.ygyno.2013.11.018

Smits, A., Lopes, A., Das, N., Bekkers, R., & Galaal, K. (2015). Quality of life in ovarian cancer survivors: The influence of obesity. *International Journal of Gynecologic Cancer, 25,* 616–621. doi:10.1097/IGC.0000000000000388

Steffen, A., Huerta, J.M., Weiderpass, E., Bueno-de-Mesquita, H.B., May, A.M., Siersema, P.D., … Boeing, H. (2015). General and abdominal obesity and risk of esophageal and gastric adenocarcinoma in the European Prospective Investigation into Cancer and Nutrition. *International Journal of Cancer, 137,* 646–657. doi:10.1002/ijc.29432

Stein, B., Anderson, J.C., Rajapakse, R., Alpern, Z.A., Messina, C.R., & Walker, G. (2010). Body mass index as a predictor of colorectal neoplasia in ethnically diverse screening population. *Digestive Diseases and Sciences, 55,* 2945–2952. doi:10.1007/s10620-009-1113-9

Stevens, V.L., Jacobs, E.J., Patel, A.V., Sun, J., Gapstur, S.M., & McCullough, M.L. (2014). Body weight in early adulthood, adult weight gain, and risk of endometrial cancer in women not using postmenopausal hormones. *Cancer Causes and Control, 25,* 321–328. doi:10.1007/s10552-013-0333-7

Tait, S., Pacheco, J.M., Gao, F., Bumb, C., Ellis, M.J., & Ma, C.X. (2014). Body mass index, diabetes, and triple-negative breast cancer prognosis. *Breast Cancer Research and Treatment, 146,* 189–197. doi:10.1007/s10549-014-3002-y

Trabert, B., Wentzensen, N., Felix, A.S., Yang, H.P., Sherman, M.E., & Brinton, L.A. (2015). Metabolic syndrome and risk of endometrial cancer in the United States: A study in the SEER-Medicare linked database. *Cancer Epidemiology, Biomarkers and Prevention, 24,* 261–267. doi:10.1158/1055-9965.EPI-14-0923

Tran, A.Q., Cohen, J.G., & Li, A.J. (2015). Impact of obesity on secondary cytoreductive surgery and overall survival in women with recurrent ovarian cancer. *Gynecologic Oncology, 138,* 263–266. doi:10.1016/j.ygyno.2015.05.035

Vance, V., Mourtzakis, M., McCargar, L., & Hanning, R. (2011). Weight gain in breast cancer survivors: Prevalence, pattern, and health consequences. *Obesity Reviews, 12,* 282–294. doi:10.1111/j.1467-789X.2010.00805.x

van Kruijsdijk, R.C.M., van der Wall, E., & Visseren, F.L.J. (2009). Obesity and cancer: The role of dysfunctional adipose tissue. *Cancer Epidemiology, Biomarkers and Prevention, 18,* 2569–2578. doi:10.1158/1055-9965.EPI-09-0372

Velanovich, V., & Szymanski, W. (1999). Quality of life of breast cancer patients with lymphedema. *American Journal of Surgery, 177,* 184–188. doi:10.1016/S0002-9610(99)00008-2

Vidal, A.C., Howard, L.E., Moreira, D.M., Castro-Santamaria, R., Andriole, G.L., Jr., & Freedland, S.J. (2014). Obesity increases the risk for high-grade prostate cancer: Results from the REDUCE study. *Cancer Epidemiology, Biomarkers and Prevention, 23,* 2936–2942. doi:10.1158/1055-9965.EPI-14-0795

Wang, L.S., Murphy, C.T., Ruth, K., Zaorsky, N.G., Smaldone, M.C., Sobczak, M.L., … Horwitz, E.M. (2015). Impact of obesity on outcomes after definitive dose–escalated intensity-modulated radiotherapy for localized prostate cancer. *Cancer, 121,* 3010–3017. doi:10.1002/cncr.29472

Wiseman, A.J., Lynch, B.M., Cameron, A.J., & Dunstan, D.W. (2014). Associations of change in television viewing time with biomarkers of postmenopausal breast cancer risk: The Australian Diabetes, Obesity, and Lifestyle Study. *Cancer Causes and Control, 25,* 1309–1319. doi:10.1007/s10552-014-0433-z

Wolin, K.Y., Luly, J., Sutcliffe, S., Andriole, G.L., & Kibel, A.S. (2010). Risk of urinary incontinence following prostatectomy: The role of physical activity and obesity. *Journal of Urology, 183,* 629–633. doi:10.1016/j.juro.2009.09.082

Wu, M.-M., Chen, H.-C., Chen, C.-L., You, S.-L., Cheng, W.-F., Chen, C.A., ... Chen, C.-J. (2014). A prospective study of gynecological cancer risk in relation to adiposity factors: Cumulative incidence and association with plasma adipokine levels. *PLOS ONE, 9*(8), e104630. doi:10.1371/journal.pone.0104630

Xu, L., Port, M., Landi, S., Gemignani, F., Cipollini, M., Elisei, R., ... Sturgis, E.M. (2014). Obesity and the risk of papillary thyroid cancer: A pooled analysis of three case-control studies. *Thyroid, 24,* 966–974. doi:10.1089/thy.2013.0566

Zhang, X., Eliassen, A.H., Tamimi, R.M., Hazra, A., Beck, A.H., Brown, M., ... Hankinson, S.E. (2015). Adult body size and physical activity in relation to risk of breast cancer according to tumor androgen receptor status. *Cancer Epidemiology, Biomarkers and Prevention, 24,* 962–968. doi:10.1158/1055-9965.EPI-14-1429

Chapter 3
Weight Management

Knowing the evidence related to the different types of diets may be useful to healthcare providers when recommending weight loss to patients. It is also useful to know what has been shown to be effective when patients ask about the "latest" diet they have read or heard about in popular media sources. A variety of weight-loss strategies have been studied in randomized trials and meta-analyses. This chapter describes the most common and popular approaches to weight loss and presents the evidence on weight loss in noncancer populations. Very little data exist in cancer populations; this is because, in part, weight loss as a side effect of treatment has been the most common issue for many patients with cancer. Therefore, many studies focus on prevention and management of cachexia. However, given the increasing evidence on the role of overweight and obesity as risk factors for cancer and cancer recurrence, attention should be paid to weight loss in overweight or obese cancer survivors and how best to encourage weight loss where appropriate.

Popular Weight-Loss Strategies

Matarese and Pories (2014) reviewed the most well-known weight-loss diets for healthy but overweight adults. These diets include low fat, very low carbohydrate, low glycemic, and the Mediterranean diet. The authors listed advantages and disadvantages of diet strategies, as well as the role of concurrent exercise and the behavioral modifications necessary for success in each approach.

Very Low Carbohydrate

Very low carbohydrate diets such as the Atkins diet (www.atkins.com) restrict carbohydrate intake to 20 g per day. In the initial, or induction, phase of the diet, restrictions are placed on the type of vegetables that can be eaten (i.e., no starchy vegetables), and no fruits, grains, pasta, bread, or legumes are permissible. The only dairy allowed is butter, cheese, and cream. Alcohol is also forbidden in the induction phase.

This phase lasts approximately two to three weeks. This is followed by the weight-loss phase, where some fruits and additional vegetables are allowed, as well as nuts, legumes, and small amounts of wine and other low-carbohydrate alcohol. This diet includes a maintenance phase and, depending on how much weight the individual wants to lose, includes the option of less restriction in daily carbohydrate intake. The Atkins diet can result in rapid initial weight loss that is highly motivating for many people. Because it has a relatively high-fat composition, dieters experience a high satiety value that may reduce total caloric intake. The low fiber composition of the diet—because of restriction of high-fiber fruits, vegetables, and grains—may result in constipation, and dieters often complain of halitosis, which is caused by the production of ketones as fat stores are broken down to produce energy.

Low Glycemic

Low-glycemic diets, such as the Zone diet (www.zonediet.com), include a mix of protein, carbohydrates, and fats in a 30%–40%–30% ratio. It claims to be an anti-inflammatory diet with a focus on low-fat protein (chicken, fish, cheese, or soy), fruits and vegetables, monounsaturated fats (olive oil, nuts, avocado), and small amounts of grains and starches. The addition of omega-3 fatty acid and polyphenol supplements is suggested to enhance the anti-inflammatory properties of the diet. Calculations of the correct proportions of the three key food groups may be taxing for some people; however, it is overall a relatively healthy diet with its focus on fruits and vegetables, low-fat proteins, and plant-based fats.

Low Fat

Low-fat diets, such as Weight Watchers, LEARN, and the Ornish diet, are also popular. Weight Watchers (www.weightwatchers.com) is probably the most well-known, with a generally balanced approach to weight loss using a points system to control caloric intake. Points are assigned to various foods based on the protein, carbohydrate, and fat content of the specific food. However, the points system can be manipulated so that dieters eat an essentially unhealthy diet but stick to the maximum number of points allowed each day. A central tenet of Weight Watchers is the support provided through in-person meetings, weigh-ins, and, more recently, online support groups and apps. Exercise and fitness is encouraged as well as emotional balance.

The LEARN diet is described as a "do it yourself" approach that focuses on lifestyle, exercise, attitudes, relationships, and nutrition. It comprises a series of 16 weekly lessons covering these concepts with eight monthly lessons thereafter. The LEARN process is taught by certified instructors, or individuals can purchase a manual that explains each lesson. The LEARN program supports other weight-loss programs such as Weight Watchers with a focus on low-fat food choices and behavior modification.

The Ornish diet, now called the Spectrum diet (http://ornishspectrum.com/proven-program/nutrition), divides food into five groups with group 1 foods being the healthiest. This group consists of fruits, vegetables, whole grains, legumes, egg whites, and nonfat dairy. Group 2 includes monounsaturated fats in the form of nuts, seeds, and avocados, with small amounts of oils permitted. Group 3 includes some seafood and other fats and oils, as well as some 2% fat dairy products and a limited number of concentrated sweeteners. Groups 4 and 5 are regarded by Ornish as the more unhealthy foods and include whole milk and full-fat dairy products, baked goods, red meat, fried foods, and processed foods. The basic concept is to eat foods that are congruent with the individual's health needs and personal values, with the idea that one should move toward the lower end of the spectrum for weight loss and health. A focus in the past of the highly restrictive Ornish diet (essentially a vegan diet) was to reverse heart disease and prevent disease. With the Spectrum approach, the emphasis is on sustainability of food choices and the recognition that foods in groups 1 and 2 will encourage weight loss and better health.

Mediterranean Diet

The Mediterranean diet focuses on eating plant-based foods (fruits and vegetables) as well as whole grains, nuts (one handful per day only), and legumes. Olive oil replaces butter and other fats, and herbs and spices should be used in place of salt for flavoring. Red meat is restricted to small portions a few times per month. A glass of red wine per day is permitted. Exercise is encouraged (45–60 minutes of daily aerobic exercise). This is one of the less restrictive diets of those described and is regarded as being heart healthy.

What Works for Weight Loss

A number of studies have compared the diets described above to assess effectiveness for various purposes, including weight loss and health-risk reduction. All of the studies and meta-analyses discussed were conducted in noncancer populations.

Dansinger and colleagues (2005) compared the Atkins, Ornish, Weight Watchers, and Zone diets in a randomized study. One hundred and sixty overweight and obese men and women were randomized to one of the four diet plans; all had been diagnosed with dyslipidemia, hypertension, or fasting hyperglycemia and ranged in age from 22 to 72. At one year, people in each of the diet groups had lost modest amounts of weight, and risk factors for cardiac disease were also moderately reduced. Adherence to the various diets was low as measured by self-report; however, those who adhered to their assigned diet reported greater weight loss and reduction of cardiac risk factors (Dansinger, Gleason, Griffith, Selker, & Schaefer, 2005).

Another study of 322 moderately obese men and women with a mean age of 52 suggested differences in adherence between men and women, with more women dropping out compared to men (29% vs. 14%; $p = 0.01$) (Greenberg, Stampfer, Schwarzfuchs, & Shai, 2009). Participants were randomized to a low-fat diet (based on guidelines from the American Heart Association, with 20%–30% of daily intake from fats), the Mediterranean diet, or the Atkins (low carbohydrate) diet. Adherence was greatest in the Atkins group but declined over time; of the participants in the Atkins group, 81% were adherent to their prescribed diet at month one. This dropped to 57% at two years. Weight loss was not significantly different by type of diet for those who were successful in keeping to the diet. Overall, the number of individuals successful in losing weight (n = 115) was less than the number of failures (n = 157). Self-reported triggers for nonadherence to the diet included holidays, with cookies (45%) and fruit (30%) being reported as the most irresistible foods. The addition of exercise was a positive factor for many; of those who exercised, 44% said they ate less after physical activity and 10% said they ate more.

Gardner et al. (2007) studied overweight premenopausal women assigned to the Atkins, Zone, Ornish, or LEARN diets compared to no dietary intervention. Women lost the most weight on a low-carbohydrate (Atkins) diet; the mean weight loss for these women at 12 months was 4.7 kg (10.36 lb) (95% confidence interval [CI] [6.3 kg, 3.1 kg]). In a meta-analysis of studies (McVay et al., 2014) comparing low-carbohydrate (Atkins, Zone, and South Beach), low-fat (Ornish), and moderate-macronutrient (Weight Watchers, Nutrisystem, Jenny Craig) diets, those on low-carbohydrate diets lost the most weight (8.73 kg [19.24 lb] at 6 months and 7.25 kg [15.98 lb] at 12 months). Those on low-fat diets lost an average of 7.99 kg (17.61 lb) at 6 months and 7.27 kg (16.02 lb) at 12 months. Little difference was noted between the individual diets in each category, but low-fat or low-carbohydrate diets appeared to result in greater weight loss than no dietary intervention. Weight loss was greatest at six months and then no more improvement was observed. Some participants even experienced some weight gain. Exercise and support enhanced weight loss. The conclusion from this meta-analysis is that women should find the program that best suits their lifestyle and offers the least barriers to adherence for them personally. McVay et al. (2014) suggested that individuals will choose a diet based on individual dietary preference and baseline food intake patterns. Therefore, the most effective recommendation may be to present patients with choices and encourage them to choose and follow the strategy that they are most comfortable with based on their usual dietary habits.

A meta-analysis comparing low-fat diets to the Mediterranean diet suggested that, at two years of follow-up, the Mediterranean diet was more effective at achieving weight loss (2.2 kg [4.85 lb]) and reducing cardiovascular risk factors (blood pressure, fasting blood glucose, total cholesterol) and inflammatory markers (C-reactive protein) (Nordmann et al., 2011).

In a study comparing low-fat with low-carbohydrate diets over two years of follow-up (Foster et al., 2010), those in the low-carbohydrate group lost approximately 11 kg (24.2 lb) at one year and 7 kg (15.4 lb) at two years for both diets. All participants received intensive behavioral interventions including weekly group sessions lasting 75–90 minutes for the first 20 weeks and then monthly for the duration of the study. Walking was required, with a goal of 50-minute walks four times per week. A low-carbohydrate diet showed greater weight loss than a low-fat diet in 200 participants, but this was not statistically significant (5.8 kg [12.7 lb] vs. 4.3 kg [9.47 lb]; $p = 0.065$). However, the low-carbohydrate diet had a greater but not statistically significant impact on cardiovascular risk factors (blood pressure, fasting blood glucose, total cholesterol) (Frisch et al., 2009).

In another study of overweight and obese adults following a three-month liquid diet, those assigned to a low-fat or low-carbohydrate diet lost weight during the maintenance phase of the study (LeCheminant et al., 2007). Alexandraki, Palacio, and Mooradian (2015) confirmed these results in their overview of low-carbohydrate versus low-fat diets. They concluded that low-carbohydrate diets result in greater weight loss at both 6 and 12 months; however, the difference in total weight loss is diminutive.

When comparing advice alone to a variety of other interventions (diet alone, diet plus exercise, exercise alone, meal replacement programs, very low calorie diets, or weight-loss medication), researchers found that reducing the amount of food consumed with the addition of exercise resulted in moderate weight loss at six months. Advice or exercise only without reducing food consumption did not have a significant effect on weight loss. The inclusion of weight-loss medications (orlistat or sibutramine) enhanced weight-loss maintenance in this study (Franz et al., 2007).

Behavioral Interventions to Promote Weight Loss

It is suggested that behavioral interventions are a positive influence on weight loss (Wadden, Butryn, Hong, & Tsai, 2014). These interventions range from face-to-face counseling to group sessions. Interventions can vary in intensity in terms of frequency and time and are offered by a range of providers including primary care physicians, dietitians, kinesiologists, nurses (including clinical nurse specialists and nurse practitioners), physician assistants, medical assistants, and health coaches. Intensive behavioral counseling by any of these providers may result in meaningful weight loss for patients. A meta-analysis of dietary counseling found that counseling resulted in a 6% net weight loss at 12 months; however, this decreased over time with weight gain seen after the initial successful weight loss up to six months, with patients returning to their baseline weight at 5.5 years (Dansinger, Tatsioni, Wong, Chung, & Balk, 2007).

A study with 141 overweight and obese adults found that adding an intensive behavioral intervention comprising group-based sessions of 60 minutes every week for the first 24 weeks and then every other week for a further 24 weeks did not show additional benefits compared to attending regular Weight Watchers meetings (Pinto, Fava, Hoffmann, & Wing, 2013).

In-person attendance at meetings and support groups may not be the best way to encourage weight loss. Access to such meetings may add additional pressure in an already busy life, and peer pressure may not always be positive, especially if weight loss does not occur for the individual. Telephone-based interventions may seem attractive; however, their value is debatable. A study comparing self-directed weight loss to either a 10- or 20-session telephone intervention found that those who completed 10 or more sessions lost more weight (5.1 kg [11.24 lb]) compared to those who participated in four or fewer sessions (0.3 kg [0.66 lb]) (Sherwood, Jeffery, Welsh, VanWormer, & Hotop, 2010). The researchers concluded that optimal timing and dose of telephone intervention are not known and should be investigated.

Interventions using cell phone methodologies (texting or instant messaging) show promise, with a net weight loss of 1.44 kg (3.17 lb) compared to controls (Liu et al., 2015). However, a study of a program using text messages to encourage lifestyle change, called LEAP (Lifestyle, Eating and Activity Program), showed that this modality can be successful (Donaldson, Fallows, & Morris, 2014). The goals of the program were to increase consumption of fruits, vegetables, and regular breakfasts and to increase daily steps taken. Participants in the study were instructed to text their progress using one message on a weekday and one message on a weekend. On receipt of the progress report, they then received a response with either praise for meeting their goals or practical tips for improvement. Compared to those in the control group who did not receive or send texts, participants lost significantly more body weight (1.6 kg [3.52 lb] vs. 0.7 kg [1.54 lb]), were less depressed, and had better quality of life.

Finally, regular self-weighing has been investigated as a strategy to increase weight loss. A systematic review of 17 studies found that weighing oneself regularly potentiates weight loss with no adverse psychological effects. More frequent weighing led to greater weight loss and less weight gain. Daily weighing appears to be optimal; however, weekly weighing is also acceptable (Zheng et al., 2015).

Mind–Body Interventions to Promote Weight Loss

Mindfulness-based interventions have been used to promote weight loss. In one study (Timmerman & Brown, 2012), 35 middle-aged women participated in six weekly sessions where education was provided on strategies to prevent weight gain when eating out; these women all ate in restaurants at least three times per week. Mindful-eating meditation was a component of the intervention. A wait-list group was used as the control group. Women who were in the intervention group ate less as measured by caloric intake, lost more weight, experienced increased diet-related self-efficacy, and reported fewer barriers to choosing food wisely when eating out.

Spirituality in African American women has been shown to prevent weight gain after an initial weight loss (Djuric et al., 2009). However, the results are modest and cannot be generalized to other populations.

Investigators have looked at whether people might be interested in using virtual technology in the form of avatars to practice weight-loss skills. In an online survey, 88% of responders said they would be interested. When the program was used in a feasibility study with eight women, 100% said they would recommend the program to others and that it played a role in their diet and exercise behaviors for the time they were using it. After four weeks, the average amount of weight lost by participating women was 1.6 kg (3.52 lb) (Napolitano et al., 2013).

Barriers and Facilitators to Weight Loss

If losing weight were a simple task, there would be few overweight or obese people, especially given what we know about the deleterious consequences of excess weight. The reality is that making choices about the foods we eat, both in quality and quantity, is difficult. It is hard to imagine that with all the messaging in the media and from health authorities, such as the Academy of Nutrition and Dietetics (www.eatright.org)

and the U.S. Department of Agriculture (www.cnpp.usda.gov/dietary-guidelines), about what constitutes a healthy diet and what foods should be avoided or rarely eaten, that the general public is not aware of what they should be doing. However, obesity has become a healthcare crisis, posing a significant risk to people of all ages.

Multiple barriers exist to weight loss, including loss of self-control and lack of self-efficacy about changing food habits, a reluctance to change eating habits, enjoyment of or craving for certain foods, lack of physical activity, life stressors prompting comfort eating, and social circumstances that promote overeating or poor food choices. Cost and access to healthy foods are also potential barriers. The list of facilitators is shorter; personal motivation, support from family and friends, and willpower are suggested as being helpful to weight loss (Hammarström, Wiklund, Lindahl, Larsson, & Ahlgren, 2014).

How a person approaches weight loss is important and may underpin the probability of success or failure, no matter the specific diet. Sairanen et al. (2014) suggested that flexibility is key; flexible control of eating has better outcomes than rigid control. Flexible control includes focusing on the present and persisting with positive behavior or change to meet the circumstances when pursuing goals of weight loss. In contrast, rigid control means that change is not possible and that adaptation to circumstances is not acceptable. Under these circumstances, people using rigid control mechanisms tend to use avoidance as a coping mechanism, and this is usually not effective (Sairanen, Lappalainen, Lapveteläinen, Tolvanen, & Karhunen, 2014).

Losing weight theoretically should increase motivation and persistence with whatever method has been chosen to achieve weight-loss goals. This is supported by a study (Baldwin, Rothman, & Jeffery, 2009) in which participants who lost weight and were satisfied with their weight loss continued to change as their bodies changed over time. Satisfaction fluctuated over time and was influenced by the amount of self-control they had to use to continue dieting, the amount of effort they exerted, and the amount of frustration they experienced. How their clothes fit was a source of satisfaction to many of the participants; this may be a useful motivator for people who are trying to lose weight and perhaps are not seeing the scale change.

Weight Loss in Cancer

Mouse studies have shown that a low-carbohydrate diet slows the growth of cancer as compared to the typical Western diet (Ho et al., 2011). However, the evidence is less strong in humans. A study that followed more than 62,000 Swedes for 17.8 years found that a moderately low carbohydrate and moderately high protein diet was not related to the incidence of cancer, regardless of the quantity of fat intake or the kind of fats consumed (Nilsson et al., 2013).

Prostate Cancer

In a small study, Ornish et al. (2005) showed that men with prostate cancer (low or intermediate risk) who were placed on a vegan diet, did moderate exercise and yoga, and attended a weekly support group saw small changes in their prostate-specific antigen levels compared to the control group. The differences in outcomes between the two groups was of uncertain clinical significance, and the protocol was intensive and may not be possible for many men.

Mavropoulos, Isaacs, Pizzo, and Freedland (2006) reviewed the data on low-carbohydrate diets in prostate cancer and concluded that a low-carbohydrate diet such as the Atkins diet may produce weight loss and lower insulin levels that are considered to play a role in cancer progression. However, the high fat component of this diet may have other deleterious effects on men's health, and the authors stopped short of endorsing it.

Breast Cancer

A number of studies have investigated the role of overweight and obesity in the breast cancer population, with far-ranging findings that support the recommendation that all women with breast cancer should be provided with information about weight management during and after treatment.

Rock et al. (2015) showed that weight loss of more than 5% of body weight had favorable effects on levels of estrone and estradiol, both of which are associated with recurrence and poor prognosis. Another study reported lower tumor necrosis factor–alpha levels, an inflammatory cytokine, in women with breast cancer who lost weight; however, the significance of this is not well established (Pakiz, Flatt, Bardwell, Rock, & Mills, 2011).

Weight loss has also been shown to lower risk for cardiovascular disease and diabetes in postmenopausal women with breast cancer (Thomson et al., 2010). In this study, an average weight loss of 6.1 kg (13.44 lb) after six months on either a low-carbohydrate or low-fat diet was seen; improvements in total/high-density lipoprotein (HDL) ratios and significant decreases in insulin and glycated hemoglobin HbA1c were observed regardless of the type of diet. The low-carbohydrate diet resulted in decreases in triglyceride levels. A diet enriched in plant-based foods and olive oil, similar to the Mediterranean diet, resulted in 80% of the breast cancer survivors losing more than 5% of total body weight over 44 weeks (Flynn & Reinert, 2010). Women who followed the olive oil–enriched diet as opposed to the National Cancer Institute diet saw higher HDL levels and lower triglyceride levels, both indicative of lower cardiovascular risk. Similar results were seen in a study of rural-dwelling women (Befort et al., 2012); fasting insulin dropped by 16.7% and leptin, an unfavorable adipocytokine, by 37.1%. Women lost an average of 14% of body weight and saw improved quality of life in the domains of sexuality, mood, and body image.

The weight gain that many women experience after treatment for breast cancer is associated with metabolic effects of treatment and lifestyle factors. Women are aware of the need to lose or maintain weight and usually know what they need to do to achieve weight loss; however, their self-efficacy may be low (Pinto et al., 2002). Rural breast cancer survivors reported a variety of psychosocial factors associated with weight gain (Befort et al., 2012). These included depression; fear of recurrence; changes in their primary relationship; alterations to body image; decreased physical strength, leading to avoidance of physical activity; and financial stress.

Interventions to promote weight loss or weight maintenance are important in this population to prevent recurrence and enhance quality of life and reduce the risk of comorbidities. Lifestyle change is possible; in a small feasibility study of African American women with breast cancer, a six-month intervention called Moving Forward was tested (Stolley, Sharp, Oh, & Schiffer, 2009). The intervention included a focus on family, music, food, social roles and relationships, and spirituality and religion. Participants made significant changes in their consumption of fatty and sweet desserts (decreased), intake of fruits and vegetables (increased), inclusion of physical exercise in daily life (increased from 0 to 24 minutes), and an increase in social support. The average weight loss was 2.5 kg (5.5 lb, 3% of body weight).

The role of endocrine manipulation in weight gain in this population is well established. Tamoxifen appears to be associated with weight gain to a greater extent than the aromatase inhibitors (Sedjo et al., 2014). In this study, women on aromatase inhibitors had a 44% reduced risk of weight gain as compared to those on tamoxifen, a selective estrogen receptor modulator. Anastrozole showed greater benefit in thinner women (body mass index [BMI] < 28 kg/m^2) (Sestak et al., 2010) than in obese women (BMI > 30 kg/m^2). The authors theorized that suppression of aromatization in adipose tissue is incomplete in obese women taking the recommended dose of 1 mg anastrozole daily. Macciò and Madeddu (2011) suggested that antidiabetic and anti-inflammatory drugs in addition to endocrine manipulation may be necessary in obese women with breast cancer.

It is recommended that until clear evidence exists on optimal weight-loss strategies for cancer survivors, regular assessment of body weight should be part of routine care throughout and after treatment. Early and individualized intervention should be recommended for survivors who are gaining weight, with the goal of a healthy weight by two years after completion of adjuvant therapy (Demark-Wahnefried et al., 2012). The American Cancer Society (ACS) has issued a series of recommendations for nutrition and physical activity during and after treatment (Doyle et al., 2006). ACS recommends common-sense approaches to weight maintenance or weight loss in the absence of cancer-specific evidence.

Encouraging Weight Loss in Patients

Factors affecting weight loss are complex and interrelated. They also are dynamic and change with life circumstances (Matarese & Pories, 2014). These include physiologic factors such as body composition (fat vs. muscle), metabolic rate, insulin sensitivity and resistance, hormones (leptin, ghrelin), and gut microbes. Age and genetics also play a role in weight loss. Social factors such as health behaviors, economic status, food supply and accessibility, and religious and cultural influences also contribute to eating patterns and diet composition.

The first step in encouraging patients to lose weight is to take a comprehensive history focused on the patient's weight, dietary history, barriers, and other considerations (see Figure 3-1). Although this may seem to be beyond the scope of healthcare provid-

Figure 3-1. Overweight- and Obesity-Focused History

Physical
- Family history of overweight and obesity
- Women: Number of pregnancies and weight gain in each
- Age at menopause if appropriate and weight change
- Medication history
- Smoking status
- Endocrine diseases (e.g., diabetes, hypothyroidism)

Behavioral
- Previous attempts at losing weight
- Dietary habits (snacking, mealtimes, fast food restaurants)
- Physical activity (type, daily amount)
- Sedentary behavior (work habits, TV watching)
- Physical limitations for exercise
- Sleep history

Social
- Living arrangements
- Social support
- Finances
- History of depression and anxiety
- Body image
- History of eating disorder(s)

Cancer History
- Type of cancer
- Treatment history
- Medication history (including adjuvant endocrine manipulation)

Note. Based on information from Kushner et al., 2013.

ers without specific education in nutrition, the components of an obesity-focused history are not dissimilar to those in any comprehensive history.

A good second step is to ask the patient to keep a food diary or journal for three days or up to a week, which can help to identify eating patterns more accurately than patient recall. The food diary should ask for details of time, place, food type and amount, and beverages consumed and should ideally include both weekdays and weekends. The diary should be reviewed with the patient and appropriate family members, especially the person responsible for buying and cooking the food that the patient eats. One of the barriers to successful weight management in the person with cancer is the role of family members who may sabotage any weight-loss efforts by the patient out of love or because they think that any weight loss is dangerous to the health of the person with cancer. This issue will be addressed in Chapter 9. A third step would be to refer the patient to a registered dietitian for expert advice and supervision. A dietitian with knowledge of cancer and its treatment would be of benefit; weight-loss attempts may not follow the usual path, and patience and understanding of the unique challenges posed by cancer are essential in working with cancer survivors.

Adolfsson and Arnold (2011) suggested a five-stage problem-solving approach to weight loss:

1. Clearly identify the problem.
   - "What do you understand about the link between overweight and obesity and risks to your health?"
   - "What part(s) of your current lifestyle is/are causing you the most problems regarding your weight?"
   - "What concerns you most about changing your present lifestyle?"
   - "What is the biggest challenge for you in relation to managing your weight?"

2. Explore feelings related to the problem.
   - "How do you feel about your weight?"
   - "How do you feel about making changes to your current lifestyle?"
   - "How will you feel if things in your life don't change?"

3. Set realistic goals to address the problem.
   - "Is it worth it for you to make some changes in your present life?"
   - "What do you think you can achieve?"
   - "What will you gain if you make changes in your life?"
   - "What do you need to do to make changes in your life?"

4. Develop a plan of action and behavior change.
   - "What do you think might work for you?"
   - "What have you tried in the past?"
   - "What worked and why?"
   - "What didn't work and why?"
   - "What do you need to get started?"

5. Evaluate the plan.
   - "What have you learned from what you tried to do?"
   - "What barriers did you encounter? How did you overcome them?"
   - "What helped you succeed?"
   - "How do you feel about what you have accomplished?"

These steps are important because the focus is patient centered; only the patients themselves will be able to affect weight loss. No matter how motivating or supportive the healthcare provider may be, it is the patient who has to make these changes.

Stages of Weight Loss

A weight loss of 5%–10% is regarded as the aim that affects metabolic risk factors and is a good starting goal (Kushner, Lawrence, & Kumar, 2013). These authors described four stages of weight loss:

1. Initial weight loss—This is a predictor for eventual total weight loss and maintenance. It may reflect adherence to the weight-loss plan, although evidence of this association is limited.
2. Plateau—Weight loss tends to occur over six months and then, despite the best adherence, most individuals find themselves at a plateau where further weight loss does not occur. This is due to a physiologic reason. Basal metabolic rate goes down and further caloric restriction or expenditure is needed to induce additional weight loss.
3. Weight-loss maintenance—This may be the most challenging stage in the weight-loss journey, where weight loss is no longer occurring and old habits may replace new ways of eating. The challenges of life events and metabolic adaptation to the new weight may lead to the regaining of weight, beginning a series of weight cycling events.
4. Weight cycling—The repeated loss and gain of weight is called *weight cycling*. Although it does not pose physical harm, in that weight gain can be followed successfully by weight loss, it may have significant psychological effects, and individuals may lose motivation to lose weight if their efforts seem to be followed by eventual weight gain.

Factors associated with weight gain include sedentary lifestyle, disinhibited eating, depression, poor coping, binge eating, emotional eating and eating in response to stress, blaming medical factors for weight gain, and passivity and wishful thinking.

Role of Healthcare Providers

Cancer diagnosis, treatment, and recovery provide teachable moments where oncology care providers have the opportunity to educate about and encourage lifestyle changes. Frontline healthcare providers are in an ideal position to start this process; however, many are not confident in their knowledge about nutrition and avoid or defer the discussion to specialists such as nutritionists (Miles, Simon, & Wardle, 2010). Rodman and Murphy (2011) suggested that nurses have limited awareness of the importance of nutrition in cancer survivorship and may not raise the topic with patients.

CASE VIGNETTE

S.K. is a 29-year-old woman who recently celebrated her one-year anniversary of her stem cell transplant for acute myeloid leukemia. Her recovery has been slow and marked by a series of complications that resulted in multiple admissions to the hospital. She is now feeling much better and has started thinking about returning to college in the fall. She had plans to attend the annual conference of Stupid Cancer, a national support and advocacy organization for young adults with cancer, but is embarrassed about the amount of weight she has gained in the months since her transplant. She explains that she does not want to go to the conference anymore because she is so ashamed of the way she looks. She says she is "fat and disgusting" and wants the nurse's advice on a diet that will help her lose at least 60 pounds over the next five months.

Questions

1. How realistic is a weight loss of 60 pounds for this young woman?
2. What advice can the nurse give her about sensible and effective weight loss specific to her stage of recovery?
3. What "red flags" should the nurse watch for in the coming weeks and months with this young woman in terms of weight loss and body image?

Conclusion

Optimal nutrition for patients with cancer is discussed in Chapter 4. Although this is important, especially during active treatment, being overweight or obese plays a significant role in cancer recurrence and the development of comorbid disease. For this reason, survivors need to manage their weight and try their best to achieve a normal and healthy weight for their age.

References

Adolfsson, B., & Arnold, M.S. (Eds.). (2011). *Behavioral approaches to treating obesity: Helping your patients make changes that last* (2nd ed.). Alexandria, VA: American Diabetes Association.

Alexandraki, I., Palacio, C., & Mooradian, A.D. (2015). Relative merits of low-carbohydrate versus low-fat diet in managing obesity. *Southern Medical Journal, 108,* 401–416. doi:10.14423/SMJ.0000000000000308

Baldwin, A.S., Rothman, A.J., & Jeffery, R.W. (2009). Satisfaction with weight loss: Examining the longitudinal covariation between people's weight-loss–related outcomes and experiences and their satisfaction. *Annals of Behavioral Medicine, 38,* 213–224. doi:10.1007/s12160-009-9148-x

Befort, C.A., Klemp, J.R., Austin, H.L., Perri, M.G., Schmitz, K.H., Sullivan, D.K., & Fabian, C.J. (2012). Outcomes of a weight loss intervention among rural breast cancer survivors. *Breast Cancer Research and Treatment, 132,* 631–639. doi:10.1007/s10549-011-1922-3

Dansinger, M.L., Gleason, J., Griffith, J.L., Selker, H.P., & Schaefer, E.J. (2005). Comparison of the Atkins, Ornish, Weight Watchers, and Zone diets for weight loss and heart disease risk reduction: A randomized trial. *JAMA, 293,* 43–53. doi:10.1001/jama.293.1.43

Dansinger, M.L., Tatsioni, A., Wong, J.B., Chung, M., & Balk, E.M. (2007). Meta-analysis: The effect of dietary counseling for weight loss. *Annals of Internal Medicine, 147,* 41–50. doi:10.7326/0003-4819-147-1-200707030-00007

Demark-Wahnefried, W., Morey, M.C., Sloane, R., Snyder, D.C., Miller, P.E., Hartman, T.J., & Cohen, H.J. (2012). Reach Out to Enhance Wellness home-based diet-exercise intervention promotes reproducible and sustainable long-term improvements in health behaviors, body weight, and physical functioning in older, overweight/obese cancer survivors. *Journal of Clinical Oncology, 30,* 2354–2361. doi:10.1200/JCO.2011.40.0895

Djuric, Z., Mirasolo, J., Kimbrough, L., Brown, D.R., Heilbrun, L.K., Canar, L., … Simon, M.S. (2009). A pilot trial of spirituality counseling for weight loss maintenance in African American breast cancer survivors. *Journal of the National Medical Association, 101,* 552–564. doi:10.1016/S0027-9684(15)30940-8

Donaldson, E.L., Fallows, S., & Morris, M. (2014). A text message based weight management intervention for overweight adults. *Journal of Human Nutrition and Dietetics, 27*(Suppl. 2), 90–97. doi:10.1111/jhn.12096

Doyle, C., Kushi, L.H., Byers, T., Courneya, K.S., Demark-Wahnefried, W., Grant, B., … Andrews, K.S. (2006). Nutrition and physical activity during and after cancer treatment: An American Cancer Society guide for informed choices. *CA: A Cancer Journal for Clinicians, 56,* 323–353. doi:10.3322/canjclin.56.6.323

Flynn, M.M., & Reinert, S.E. (2010). Comparing an olive oil–enriched diet to a standard lower-fat diet for weight loss in breast cancer survivors: A pilot study. *Journal of Women's Health, 19,* 1155–1161. doi:10.1089/jwh.2009.1759

Foster, G.D., Wyatt, H.R., Hill, J.O., Makris, A.P., Rosenbaum, D.L., Brill, C., … Klein, S. (2010). Weight and metabolic outcomes after 2 years on a low-carbohydrate versus low-fat diet: A randomized trial. *Annals of Internal Medicine, 153,* 147–157. doi:10.7326/0003-4819-153-3-201008030-00005

Franz, M.J., VanWormer, J.J., Crain, A.L., Boucher, J.L., Histon, T., Caplan, W., … Pronk, N.P. (2007). Weight-loss outcomes: A systematic review and meta-analysis of weight-loss clinical trials with a minimum 1-year follow-up. *Journal of the American Dietetic Association, 107,* 1755–1767. doi:10.1016/j.jada.2007.07.017

Frisch, S., Zittermann, A., Berthold, H.K., Götting, C., Kuhn, J., Kleesiek, K., … Körtke, H. (2009). A randomized controlled trial on the efficacy of carbohydrate-reduced or fat-reduced diets in patients attending a telemedically guided weight loss program. *Cardiovascular Diabetology, 8,* 36. doi:10.1186/1475-2840-8-36

Gardner, C.D., Kiazand, A., Alhassan, S., Kim, S., Stafford, R.S., Balise, R.R., … King, A.C. (2007). Comparison of the Atkins, Zone, Ornish, and LEARN diets for change in weight and related risk factors among overweight premenopausal women: The A to Z weight loss study: A randomized trial. *JAMA, 297,* 969–977. doi:10.1001/jama.297.9.969

Greenberg, I., Stampfer, M.J., Schwarzfuchs, D., & Shai, I. (2009). Adherence and success in long-term weight loss diets: The Dietary Intervention Randomized Controlled Trial (DIRECT). *Journal of the American College of Nutrition, 28,* 159–168. doi:10.1080/07315724.2009.10719767

Hammarström, A., Wiklund, A.F., Lindahl, B., Larsson, C., & Ahlgren, C. (2014). Experiences of barriers and facilitators to weight-loss in a diet intervention—A qualitative study of women in northern Sweden. *BMC Women's Health, 14,* 59. doi:10.1186/1472-6874-14-59

Ho, V.W., Leung, K., Hsu, A., Luk, B., Lai, J., Shen, S.Y., … Krystal, G. (2011). A low carbohydrate, high protein diet slows tumor growth and prevents cancer initiation. *Cancer Research, 71,* 4484–4493. doi:10.1158/0008-5472.CAN-10-3973

Kushner, R., Lawrence, V., & Kumar, S. (2013). *Practical manual of clinical obesity.* Hoboken, NJ: Wiley-Blackwell.

LeCheminant, J.D., Gibson, C.A., Sullivan, D.K., Hall, S., Washburn, R., Vernon, M.C., … Donnelly, J.E. (2007). Comparison of a low carbohydrate and low fat diet for weight maintenance in overweight or obese adults enrolled in a clinical weight management program. *Nutrition Journal, 6,* 36. doi:10.1186/1475-2891-6-36

Liu, F., Kong, X., Cao, J., Chen, S., Li, C., Huang, J., … Kelly, T.N. (2015). Mobile phone intervention and weight loss among overweight and obese adults: A meta-analysis of randomized controlled trials. *American Journal of Epidemiology, 181,* 337–348. doi:10.1093/aje/kwu260

Macciò, A., & Madeddu, C. (2011). Obesity, inflammation, and postmenopausal breast cancer: Therapeutic implications. *Scientific World Journal, 11,* 2020–2036. doi:10.1100/2011/806787

Matarese, L.E., & Pories, W.J. (2014). Adult weight loss diets: Metabolic effects and outcomes. *Nutrition in Clinical Practice, 29,* 759–767. doi:10.1177/0884533614550251

Mavropoulos, J.C., Isaacs, W.B., Pizzo, S.V., & Freedland, S.J. (2006). Is there a role for a low-carbohydrate ketogenic diet in the management of prostate cancer? *Urology, 68,* 15–18. doi:10.1016/j.urology.2006.03.073

McVay, M.A., Voils, C.I., Coffman, C.J., Geiselman, P.J., Kolotkin, R.L., Mayer, S.B., ... Yancy, W.S., Jr. (2014). Factors associated with choice of a low-fat or low-carbohydrate diet during a behavioral weight loss intervention. *Appetite, 83,* 117–124. doi:10.1016/j.appet.2014.08.023

Miles, A., Simon, A., & Wardle, J. (2010). Answering patient questions about the role lifestyle factors play in cancer onset and recurrence. *Journal of Health Psychology, 15,* 291–298. doi:10.1177/1359105309351245

Napolitano, M.A., Hayes, S., Russo, G., Muresu, D., Giordano, A., & Foster, G.D. (2013). Using avatars to model weight loss behaviors: Participant attitudes and technology development. *Journal of Diabetes Science and Technology, 7,* 1057–1065. doi:10.1177/193229681300700430

Nilsson, L.M., Winkvist, A., Johansson, I., Lindahl, B., Hallmans, G., Lenner, P., & Van Guelpen, B. (2013). Low-carbohydrate, high-protein diet score and risk of incident cancer: A prospective cohort study. *Nutrition Journal, 12,* 58. doi:10.1186/1475-2891-12-58

Nordmann, A.J., Suter-Zimmermann, K., Bucher, H.C., Shai, I., Tuttle, K.R., Estruch, R., & Briel, M. (2011). Meta-analysis comparing Mediterranean to low-fat diets for modification of cardiovascular risk factors. *American Journal of Medicine, 124,* 841–851. doi:10.1016/j.amjmed.2011.04.024

Ornish, D., Weidner, G., Fair, W.R., Marlin, R., Pettengill, E.B., Raisin, C.J., ... Carroll, P.R. (2005). Intensive lifestyle changes may affect the progression of prostate cancer. *Journal of Urology, 174,* 1065–1070. doi:10.1097/01.ju.0000169487.49018.73

Pakiz, B., Flatt, S.W., Bardwell, W.A., Rock, C.L., & Mills, P.J. (2011). Effects of a weight loss intervention on body mass, fitness, and inflammatory biomarkers in overweight or obese breast cancer survivors. *International Journal of Behavioral Medicine, 18,* 333–341. doi:10.1007/s12529-010-9079-8

Pinto, A.M., Fava, J.L., Hoffmann, D.A., & Wing, R.R. (2013). Combining behavioral weight loss treatment and a commercial program: A randomized clinical trial. *Obesity, 21,* 673–680. doi:10.1002/oby.20044

Pinto, B.M., Maruyama, N.C., Clark, M.M., Cruess, D.G., Park, E., & Roberts, M. (2002). Motivation to modify lifestyle risk behaviors in women treated for breast cancer. *Mayo Clinic Proceedings, 77,* 122–129. doi:10.4065/77.2.122

Rock, C.L., Flatt, S.W., Byers, T.E., Colditz, G.A., Demark-Wahnefried, W., Ganz, P.A., ... Wyatt, H. (2015). Results of the Exercise and Nutrition to Enhance Recovery and Good Health for You (ENERGY) Trial: A behavioral weight loss intervention in overweight or obese breast cancer survivors. *Journal of Clinical Oncology, 33,* 3169–3176. doi:10.1200/JCO.2015.61.1095

Rodman, S.R., & Murphy, J.L. (2011). Nutrition knowledge and attitudes of pre-registered and registered nurses in relation to cancer survivorship. *Proceedings of the Nutrition Society, 70.* doi:10.1017/S0029665111003922

Sairanen, E., Lappalainen, R., Lapveteläinen, A., Tolvanen, A., & Karhunen, L. (2014). Flexibility in weight management. *Eating Behaviors, 15,* 218–224. doi:10.1016/j.eatbeh.2014.01.008

Sedjo, R.L., Byers, T., Ganz, P.A., Colditz, G.A., Demark-Wahnefried, W., Wolin, K.Y., ... Rock, C.L. (2014). Weight gain prior to entry into a weight-loss intervention study among overweight and obese breast cancer survivors. *Journal of Cancer Survivorship, 8,* 410–418. doi:10.1007/s11764-014-0351-9

Sestak, I., Distler, W., Forbes, J.F., Dowsett, M., Howell, A., & Cuzick, J. (2010). Effect of body mass index on recurrences in tamoxifen and anastrozole treated women: An exploratory analysis from the ATAC Trial. *Journal of Clinical Oncology, 28,* 3411–3415. doi:10.1200/JCO.2009.27.2021

Sherwood, N.E., Jeffery, R.W., Welsh, E.M., VanWormer, J., & Hotop, A.M. (2010). The Drop It At Last Study: Six-month results of a phone-based weight loss trial. *American Journal of Health Promotion, 24,* 378–383. doi:10.4278/ajhp.080826-QUAN-161

Stolley, M.R., Sharp, L.K., Oh, A., & Schiffer, L. (2009). A weight loss intervention for African American breast cancer survivors, 2006. *Prevention of Chronic Disease, 6,* A22. Retrieved from https://www.cdc.gov/pcd/issues/2009/jan/08_0026.htm

Thomson, C.A., Stopeck, A.T., Bea, J.W., Cussler, E., Nardi, E., Frey, G., & Thompson, P.A. (2010). Changes in body weight and metabolic indexes in overweight breast cancer survivors enrolled in a randomized trial of low-fat vs. reduced carbohydrate diets. *Nutrition and Cancer, 62,* 1142–1152. doi:10.1080/01635581.2010.513803

Timmerman, G.M., & Brown, A. (2012). The effect of a mindful restaurant eating intervention on weight management in women. *Journal of Nutrition Education and Behavior, 44,* 22–28. doi:10.1016/j.jneb.2011.03.143

Wadden, T.A., Butryn, M.L., Hong, P.S., & Tsai, A.G. (2014). Behavioral treatment of obesity in patients encountered in primary care settings: A systematic review. *JAMA, 312,* 1779–1791. doi:10.1001/jama.2014.14173

Zheng, Y., Klem, M.L., Sereika, S.M., Danford, C.A., Ewing, L.J., & Burke, L.E. (2015). Self-weighing in weight management: A systematic literature review. *Obesity, 23,* 256–265. doi:10.1002/oby.20946

Chapter 4
Optimal Nutrition

Although the focus of this book is on reducing overweight and obesity in cancer survivors, it is important to know what constitutes optimal nutrition for cancer survivors before, during, and after treatment. Cancer survivors are sometimes told a number of myths by well-meaning friends and family members. They may hear or read claims in the media about foods to avoid (for example, sugar) and supplements that can cure cancer. This chapter presents what we know about optimal nutrition for cancer survivors. Oncology care providers need to know the evidence about these claims and advice in order to guide and educate their patients to eat as well as possible to both lose weight and maintain a healthy weight to promote healing from treatment and overall good health.

Cancer Treatment and Its Influence on Optimal Nutrition

Surgery

All of the therapies used in treating cancer have the potential to affect patients' ability to eat a healthy diet. Surgery—especially to the gastrointestinal tract, beginning with the mouth and ending with the rectum and anus—will affect not only food choices but also the ability of the body to metabolize and use the nutrients in the food that is eaten. Weight loss is common in the days and weeks following surgery when the patient may not be able to buy, prepare, and cook nutritious food. Family and friends often are more than willing to help, but not all patients may have supportive people around them who can help.

Suggestions for maintaining adequate intake after surgery include bland foods that are easy to digest. High-fat foods should be avoided and care should be taken to include lean protein to promote wound healing. Small, frequent meals are preferable to larger meals, and patients should be encouraged to eat when hungry instead of waiting for their usual mealtimes. This can put strain on family members who are used to eating at identified times and may find that they have to work hard to meet the needs or demands of someone recovering from surgery and wanting frequent snacks. Fresh fruits and vegetables as well as dairy products contain vitamins and minerals important for wound healing.

Adequate fluid intake is also important. Patients may avoid adequate fluid intake, especially in the early days after surgery when getting up and walking to and from the bathroom may be painful.

Radiation

The same advice for small, healthy meals eaten frequently throughout the day applies to patients undergoing radiation. One of the challenges of radiation therapy is that it is usually given over extended periods of time; therefore, patients may be away from home for parts of the day and find maintaining their food and fluid intake challenging. Patients who live far from the treatment center may stay in hotels or hostels close to where their treatment occurs and may have limited access to grocery stores, a kitchen, or even a refrigerator to store and prepare foods. They may find that they have to buy fast food or eat packaged snacks and meals that are high in salt, sugar, and fat.

Radiation to the gastrointestinal tract may cause nausea, making eating and drinking difficult. Attention to controlling these side effects is very important in maintaining optimal nutrition. Fatigue also is very common during and after radiation therapy. This can affect patients' appetite as well as their ability to prepare healthy foods.

Chemotherapy

Because of the systemic side effects of chemotherapy, nutritional balance can easily be affected. From stomatitis to nausea and vomiting, it is not uncommon for patients to lose weight during treatment. Some patients, however, will experience weight gain if they are on concomitant steroids to manage side effects. Fatigue also is common, and keeping well-hydrated and eating small amounts of calorie- and protein-rich foods can help patients maintain weight and mitigate their fatigue.

Endocrine Therapy

Commonly used to treat breast and prostate cancer, endocrine therapies often cause unwanted weight gain that can be difficult to lose; many patients are prescribed these therapies for extended periods of time. Managing portion size and learning to eat less may be necessary to maintain weight, even if weight loss is not possible. Although important for all cancer survivors, incorporating physical activity becomes even more important for individuals on these medications, as they have to somehow tip the "calories in versus calories out" balance in favor of using more energy than calories consumed (Grant, Bloch, Hamilton, & Thomson, 2010).

Weight Loss During Treatment

It is not uncommon for individuals to lose weight during treatment. This can be a mixed blessing, with some patients enjoying being "thin" for the first time in their adult lives. However, caution should be taken to ensure that the weight loss is not too severe, as it can cause immune suppression, fatigue, lengthened and complicated recovery, and decreased quality of life.

Weight loss during treatment can pose a danger to patients who begin treatment underweight, and healthcare providers should be able to advise patients if they are losing weight consistently throughout treatment. A number of strategies exist to increase calorie intake without increasing the amount of food ingested, including the following:

- Adding high-fat cheese and other dairy products to the diet
- Increasing the number of eggs eaten daily
- Eating dried fruits as a snack
- Adding breading to oven-baked protein
- Adding nonfat dried milk to soups and smoothies
- Adding nuts and seeds to the diet
- Ensuring that high-quality protein is eaten with every meal

Weight loss during treatment carries some social stigma as well, with patients being identified as having cancer because of their sudden weight loss and resultant gaunt appearance. This can be distressing for patients and their families and may lead to isolation if individuals are too embarrassed to go out in public.

Myths and Misinformation

It is not uncommon for well-meaning friends, family, colleagues, and strangers to offer cancer survivors advice about nutrition. These are often not based on fact and usually come from short articles in magazines and other media. As discussed in other chapters in this book, cancer survivors often feel that they have little control over what has happened to them, and doing something about what they eat seems like the only thing they can control. Therefore, it is easy to see how avoiding certain foods or using dietary supplements seems to make sense. A lot of myths and misinformation exist that, at best, are useless but may in fact be harmful to survivors.

Sugar

One of these harmful ideas is that sugar feeds cancer, and any and all sugars, including fruits, should be avoided. No evidence exists to support this. In fact, avoiding natural sugars, such as those found in fruits and vegetables, may be deleterious to the health of cancer survivors. Eating the recommended five servings of fruits and vegetables per day provides fiber, vitamins, water, and antioxidants. Avoiding refined sugar, especially those in high-fat snacks and commercial-baked goods, is another matter; these foods tend to be high in calories and preservatives and may cause weight gain or at least an inability to lose or maintain weight at a healthy level.

Alcohol

Alcohol generally should be consumed with caution. Alcohol is associated with a risk for hepatic, oropharyngeal, esophageal, breast, gastric, and colorectal cancers; however, no evidence to date supports a link between alcohol and cancer recurrence.

Organic Foods

Many cancer survivors choose to move to an organic food diet after diagnosis. To be labeled and sold as organic, food must be certified by the U.S. Department of Agriculture (USDA). Organic farming does not use synthetic fertilizers, sewage, irradiation, or genetic engineering (USDA, 2016). Organic foods are not necessarily more nutritious, but the absence of these aforementioned farming practices may have benefits. They are usually eaten closer to harvest because they deteriorate more rapidly than nonorganic foods. Organic foods usually are more expensive and may not be available in smaller cities and towns. The usual practices for safe food handling should be followed, including handwashing and washing of all produce, as even organic foods can contain dirt, insects, and stray residue from fertilizers and insecticides.

Special Diet Regimens

Some believe that special diet regimens exist that can help to remove toxins from the body during cancer treatment or that can cure or treat cancer. No scientific evidence supports these claims, and a full description and analysis of these regimens can be found in the American Cancer Society's (ACS's) *Complete Guide to Complementary and Alternative Cancer Therapies*. Examples of such diets include Livingston-Wheeler Therapy (which claims to increase immunity) and metabolic therapies such as Gerson Therapy, Kelley's Treatment, and the Gonzalez Regimen.

Some patients with cancer choose to avoid animal products and adopt a vegetarian diet, a macrobiotic diet, or include juicing and fasting in their diets. Evidence is limited that a vegetarian diet will reduce the risk of developing some cancers, and no evidence exists that any of these regimens can cure cancer. Fasting introduces additional risks to patients already at risk for weight loss, and juicing removes essential fiber from fruits and vegetables. ACS encourages a mostly plant-based diet with limited red meat and processed foods (Grant et al., 2010).

What Is the Optimal Food Plan for Cancer Survivors?

Several organizations have developed dietary recommendations and resources that healthcare providers can use to guide patients (see Table 4-1). Referral to a nutritionist may be necessary for some patients.

ACS recommends the following as the optimal diet for cancer survivors:

- Limit consumption of red and processed meat.
- Eat at least 2.5 cups of fresh fruit and vegetables daily.
- Choose whole grains instead of refined grains.
- Limit consumption of alcoholic beverages to one per day for women and two per day for men.

These recommendations are similar to the 2015–2020 dietary guidelines issued by the U.S. Department of Health and Human Services and USDA (DeSalvo, Olson, & Casavale, 2016):

- Consume a variety of vegetables, including dark green, red, and orange vegetables.
- Consume a variety of beans and legumes.
- Consume starchy vegetables.

Table 4-1. Resources

Organization	Resources
Academy of Nutrition and Dietetics www.eatright.org	Information on nutrition and reference materials
American Cancer Society www.cancer.org	Information for people with cancer including dietary information
Cancer.Net www.cancer.net/survivorship	Life changes after cancer
Centers for Disease Control and Prevention www.cdc.gov/cancer/survivorship	General information and support for caregivers
Physicians Committee for Responsible Medicine www.pcrm.org	Healthy eating tips and recipes written by physicians and dietitians
World Cancer Research Fund International http://wcrf.org/int/research-we-fund/continuous-update-project-cup	Expert panel review of diet, exercise, and risk reduction research

- Consume whole fruits.
- Consume grains, with at least half of these being whole grains.
- Consume fat-free or low-fat dairy products and/or fortified soy beverages.
- Consume a variety of proteins, including fish and seafood, lean meats and poultry, eggs, legumes, nuts, seeds, and soy products.
- Cook with some oils (e.g., olive oil or other vegetable oils).
- Limit amount of added sugar (less than 10% of daily calorie total).
- Limit amount of saturated fats (less than 10% of daily calorie total).
- Limit sodium intake to less than 2,300 mg daily.
- Consume alcohol in moderation: One drink per day for women and two per day for men.

As described in Chapter 5, 150 minutes of moderate-intensity physical activity per week also is recommended for cancer survivors. A number of useful resources are available to oncology care providers to help guide patients (see Table 4-1).

CASE VIGNETTE

J.B. is a 67-year-old man recently diagnosed with low-risk prostate cancer. On the advice of his urologist, he goes on active surveillance to monitor the status of the cancer and to avoid surgery or radiation for as long as possible. Although he is satisfied with this treatment option, his wife and grown child are not.

His 38-year-old daughter, C.B., calls the clinic repeatedly asking for guidance on his diet. She read about foods that J.B. should include and avoid in his diet that will help "cure the cancer." C.B. is terrified that her father is going to die because of his decision to not have surgery immediately and wants to do everything in her power to prevent this from happening.

C.B.'s list of "forbidden" foods is long: all sugar, alcohol, all fruits, starchy vegetables, and all animal proteins. C.B. has been forcing her father to drink kale smoothies for breakfast every day and eat a salad with 2 oz of skinless chicken breast for both lunch and dinner and no snacks.

Questions

1. How should the nurse deal with this situation without alienating C.B.?
2. Where should the nurse look for the best evidence on diet and cancer?
3. Do C.B.'s food choices for her father sound like a good idea?

In this case, a discussion that incorporates the Ask-Tell-Ask approach may be helpful for J.B., his wife, and his daughter (see Chapter 7).

Ask

Nurse: J.B., your daughter obviously cares about you very much and is doing what she thinks is right for you. How do you feel about the nutritional regimen she has you on, and what information do you need or want in this regard?

J.B.: I've lost seven pounds since I was here two weeks ago, and I'm starving all the time. I'm still working, and I just don't have the energy to do what I have to do. There are days when I think I should just have the surgery so at least I can go back to eating the way I used to!

J.B.'s wife: Honey, C.B. is just trying to do her best for you.

C.B.: Dad, this is important to me, to all of us! I want you to be healthy. And everything I read says that you need to control your diet.

Tell

Nurse: Let's just take a step back. C.B., I know you want what is best for your dad, and you obviously love him very much. However, a lot of what you are telling him to do has no basis in evidence. Your dad has lost a significant amount of weight, and this is affecting his daily activities. He should not be hungry every day. He should be eating lean protein and lots of fruits and vegetables, but the restrictive diet you have put him on is not doing him any good. He was not overweight to begin with, and he should not lose any more weight. I am going to make an appointment for J.B. to see a nutritionist who works with our clinic, and I want you ALL to go and meet her.

J.B.: Thank you! I'll meet this nutritionist, just for the chance of C.B. learning that this diet is nuts!

J.B.'s wife: I would like to know more about how to support you with this active surveillance thing, and perhaps we can all eat better.

Ask

Nurse: That's great. In the meantime, here is a booklet with advice and suggestions from the American Cancer Society. It has some recipes in the back, too, and is based on the best available evidence. Is there anything else I can tell you or any other issues you would like me to address today?

Conclusion

A healthy diet has been linked to the prevention of certain cancers; however, not everyone has eaten well for all of their lives. For cancer survivors, eating well is associated with general well-being and potentially lowering the risk for recurrence and the development of secondary cancers. However, diet is not the only risk factor. While survivors may be tempted to radically change their diets in response to their diagnosis, a common-sense approach is the most appropriate. Following ACS's recommendations is one such approach that has been studied and supported by evidence. No special diet or program exists that can prevent, cure, or otherwise alter the course of disease or the body's response to treatment.

References

DeSalvo, K.B., Olson, R., & Casavale, K.O. (2016). Dietary guidelines for Americans. *JAMA, 135,* 457–458. doi:10.1001/jama.2015.18396

Grant, B.L., Bloch, A.S., Hamilton, K.K., & Thomson, C.A. (Eds.). (2010). *American Cancer Society complete guide to nutrition for cancer survivors: Eating well, staying well during and after cancer care* (2nd ed.). Atlanta, GA: American Cancer Society.

U.S. Department of Agriculture. (2016). Organic production and handling standards. Retrieved from https://www.ams.usda.gov/publications/content/organic-production-handling-standards

Chapter 5
Physical Activity and Weight Management

Over the past decade, an increasing number of studies have been published that support the role of physical activity and exercise in the lives of cancer survivors at all stages of the cancer trajectory. Physical activity also is recommended as an effective way of managing weight, especially when combined with reduction in calorie intake. However, exercise is not part of every cancer survivor's daily life. Many of the studies published focus on interventions to promote and encourage survivors to start some kind of exercise and then maintain it over a year or more. For most people, incorporating physical activity in daily life means finding the motivation to start and then continue that level of activity. This is one of the biggest challenges for many. This chapter will describe the research on physical activity and body weight and the programs and interventions focused on exercise and weight loss. It will also describe how individuals can increase their motivation to include daily physical activity and exercise and offers suggestions for oncology care providers to assist in helping survivors in integrating physical activity and exercise into their lives.

Physical Activity and Quality of Life

Incorporation of physical activity and exercise improves general quality of life, supports return to work, mitigates fatigue and depression, and aids in weight loss and weight-loss maintenance (Fong et al., 2012). It also has direct benefits on psychological and social health and plays a role in short- and long-term adaptation and recovery and overall quality of life (Burke & Utley, 2013; Voskuil et al., 2010).

The American College of Sports Medicine (Schmitz et al., 2010) concluded that exercise during and after treatment for cancer is safe and results in improved quality of life, cancer-related fatigue, and physical functioning for cancer survivors. The College also recommended following the 2008 Physical Activity Guidelines for Americans (150 minutes of moderate-intensity exercise per week) with adaptations if necessary due to adverse effects of treatment (U.S. Department of Health and Human Services, 2008).

Although most of the studies on physical activity and exercise and cancer are conducted in women with breast cancer, a limited number of studies involve individuals with other kinds of cancer. Many of the intervention studies include both physical activity and diet, following the predominant paradigm that a combination will increase weight loss.

Breast Cancer

As with many other areas of interest in cancer survivorship, studies in women with breast cancer dominate the available evidence. Studies have been conducted in women during active treatment, in the post-treatment phase, and into long-term survivorship. Many women begin their breast cancer trajectory with poor physical activity levels. In one study, just 12% of the women met the criteria for regular exercise at high intensity; the vast majority (65%) performed only low-intensity physical activity (Mohammadi, Sulaiman, Koon, Amani, & Hosseini, 2013). Overweight and obese breast cancer survivors are known to experience more pain than breast cancer survivors of a normal weight. Women who meet the target for physical activity are also less likely to report pain (Forsythe et al., 2013). Physical activity has been shown to mitigate a variety of side effects of adjuvant therapy, including depression, fatigue, weight gain, loss of muscle strength, and decreased quality of life (Loprinzi & Cardinal, 2012); this has been shown in premenopausal women, too (Hojan, Molińska-Glura, & Milecki, 2013).

Women in Active Treatment

A small study of women treated with chemotherapy who participated in a structured physical activity intervention at a rehabilitation hospital found multiple benefits (Backman, Browall, Sundberg, & Wengström, 2015). The women felt more confident exercising in a rehabilitation facility where there were others who had lost hair due to treatment. They saw exercise as having physical and functional benefits in terms of increased energy initially and improvements in other side effects of chemotherapy such as dizziness and shortness of breath. However, as their exposure to chemotherapy increased with cumulative treatment, many found it more difficult to participate in the exercise program. Overall, the women saw physical exercise as a way of maintaining their initial physical health and helping them to recover from the effects of chemotherapy; it also allowed them to feel normal and independent instead of playing the "cancer patient" role.

Another study of women in active treatment used motivational interviewing and social cognitive theory to evaluate whether women on treatment could comply with a healthy lifestyle program (Djuric et al., 2011). The program included a low-fat diet high in fruits and vegetables with moderate exercise. Seventy-five percent of those recruited into the study completed 12 months on the program and were satisfied with their participation. The women were randomized to receive either written material (controls) or telephone counseling. The findings of the study suggested that weight gain may be prevented in women on chemotherapy, an issue that is concerning to many women with breast cancer. Body weight and diet are sources of personal vulnerability for some women, and participating in physical exercise may be a way to regain some control (Maley, Warren, & Devine, 2013). The women in this study reported that exercise was not only a way to deal with the excess weight they had gained, but it also helped them to manage stress. For some women, during the acute treatment phase when they could not exercise as they normally did, this was experienced as another loss related to diagnosis.

A small study in Korea found that a 12-week walking program for women receiving chemotherapy resulted in significant weight loss, loss of body fat, and change in body mass index (Kim, Shin, & Suk, 2015). The women in this study walked for 30–40 minutes at moderate intensity five days per week.

Myths related to physical activity while undergoing active treatment include patients believing that they cannot exercise because they need to conserve their energy for dealing with the treatment regimen (Loh, Chew, & Lee, 2011). Women who do not meet the guidelines for physical activity may experience poorer quality of life; being obese is associated with poorer physical functioning. African American women tend to fall into this category with higher levels of obesity and lower levels of physical activity (Paxton et al., 2012).

Exercise may be seen as a way of preparing to live a healthier life after breast cancer (Bulmer, Howell, Ackerman, & Fedric, 2012). The benefits of increased stamina and strength gained with incorporating exercise into daily routine were surprising to women in another study (Balneaves et al., 2014). This was paradoxical in that they thought they would lose weight—which they did not—and yet, they felt better psychologically and felt stronger and more in control. Women may use exercise as a way of dealing with their weight gain and changed body after treatment (Brunet, Burke, & Sabiston, 2013); however, their ability to do so may be affected by long-term and late effects of treatment such as lymphedema, peripheral neuropathy, fatigue, and insomnia. The association between exercise and weight loss appears ubiquitous among breast cancer survivors, including those up to age 86 in one study (Whitehead & Lavelle, 2009).

Women After Active Treatment

Multiple factors influence weight gain during treatment and weight maintenance or loss when treatment is over. One of the factors is whether breast cancer survivors return to work after treatment. Working status appears to play a role in whether women with breast cancer are able to be physically active (Charlier et al., 2012). In one study, women who were not working reported fatigue and body image issues as factors leading to physical inactivity. Working women reported the effects of chemotherapy and upper limb problems as barriers, but headaches, feeling unwell, and poor body image were motivators to including physical activity in their daily lives.

Women who gain weight over the first two years after a breast cancer diagnosis are at higher risk of limitations in their physical functioning, which may affect their ability to participate in physical exercise. In a large study of breast cancer survivors, those who gained more than 10% of their prediagnosis weight were twice as likely to report functional limitations (Young et al., 2014). Overweight or obese women with breast cancer participated in a 12-week study with a lifestyle intervention that included a low-calorie diet with intensive weekly educational sessions led by a dietitian and twice-weekly sessions of aerobic and resistance exercise lasting 75 minutes and supervised by exercise specialists (Travier et al., 2014). Participants in the program lost a significant amount of weight (5.6 ± 2 kg) over the 12-week period; however, whether this was maintained over time was not assessed.

Weight loss and bone density were maintained in a small study of women with breast cancer who participated in a 16- to 24-week supervised walking intervention. Maintaining bone density is an important consideration for postmenopausal women at risk for osteoporosis, and this intervention, provided at community fitness centers, was feasible with high adherence in the small sample (Knobf, Insogna, DiPietro, Fennie, & Thompson, 2008). A randomized trial of three-times-weekly moderate-intensity resistance and impact exercise in breast cancer survivors showed that the intervention preserved bone density compared to the control group, who did low-intensity stretching (Winters-Stone et al., 2011). This reduced the risk of fractures. The authors concluded that this was particularly important for women on aromatase inhibitors because muscle mass increased, which is associated with a lower risk of falls.

Although studies such as the ones described in this chapter usually measure weight loss and physical fitness, Scott et al. (2013) also measured cardiopulmonary fitness and cardiovascular function in a sample of 90 breast cancer survivors. The women participated in a six-month lifestyle intervention comprising three exercise classes per week, individual dietary advice, and weekly nutrition seminars. Although those who were in the intervention arm experienced just a modest amount of weight loss, central adiposity (measured by waist circumference) was reduced significantly, and improvements in cardiopulmonary fitness and cardiovascular function were seen. Positive effects on risk factors were also observed in a three-month adapted physical activity program, particularly among sedentary survivors who were spending more than nine hours each day either sitting or lying down (Foucaut et al., 2014).

Women with triple-negative breast cancer are known to have a poorer prognosis. Healthy eating and physical activity have shown benefit in this high-risk population, including weight loss (mainly from loss of fat), improved quality of life, and decreased sedentary time (Swisher et al., 2015).

Minority Women

Little is known about what, if any, differences in attitudes to weight loss are influenced by culture and ethnicity. African American women are known to be more obese in general compared to Caucasian women and have lower physical activity levels (Sheppard et al., 2016). In a study of obese African American breast cancer survivors, participants lost very little weight (0.8% of body weight) after a 12-week intervention that included education about nutrition, exercise in a group format, and telephone sessions using motivational interviewing techniques (see Chapter 8). The intervention used culturally sensitive approaches, including content related to spirituality, faith, body image perception, and traditional foods. Despite this, the women did not reach the targeted 5% weight loss. Conducting interventions for African American women in a community setting has been shown to be feasible and may improve quality of life and even overall survival (Nock et al., 2015).

Interventions Promoting Physical Activity

Programs to test the effectiveness of physical activity and various outcomes usually include a nutritional outcome. This complies with the perspective that weight loss cannot be achieved or maintained without this dual approach.

A six-month intervention including three supervised exercise sessions per week with individual diet advice and group nutrition seminars showed positive results with improved cardiopulmonary fitness and quality of life for those who participated in the intervention as compared to those in a control group (Scott et al., 2013). Another study of a short-term diet and physical activity intervention (12 weeks in duration) comprised twice-weekly supervised exercise sessions with weekly nutrition group sessions. Participants experienced decreased fatigue and improved quality-of-life scores in addition to weight loss (Travier et al., 2014).

The ENERGY trial (Exercise and Nutrition to Enhance Recovery and Good Health for You) (Demark-Wahnefried et al., 2015; Rock et al., 2015) randomized breast cancer survivors to an intensive group-based intervention or a less intensive control group. The study took place over two years. During this time, the intervention group lost more than three times the weight of the control group (6% vs. 1.5% of initial weight), but physical activity levels were less favorable. At the 6- and 12-month interval, women in the intervention group participated in exercise more than the control group (238 women and 212 minutes per week in the intervention group compared to 163 women and 139 minutes per week in the control group). At the 18- and 24-month interval, both groups were similar in the amount of time spent in physical activity (168 women and 165 minutes per week for the intervention group compared to 158 women and 157 minutes per week for the control group).

Commercial weight-loss programs may be appealing to women after breast cancer, as the programs are widely advertised and available in their communities. Greenlee et al. (2013) conducted a randomized trial of the Curves Complete weight-loss program in a sample of minority women (Hispanic, African American, and African Caribbean). Compared to the control group, those who participated in the program (30 minutes of exercise in a circuit with a low-fat, high-vegetable, calorie-restricted diet) lost more weight (3.3% compared to 1.8%); however, some of this weight was regained over a six-month period.

Including family members in being more physically active may have benefits for them as well as for the cancer survivor. Anton, Partridge, and Morrissy (2013) found that family caregivers experienced improved psychological and physical well-being, were able to offer tangible support to their loved one with cancer, and experienced support for themselves by participating in a program for survivors and their caregivers.

Dragon boat racing is a unique form of exercise that is popular with breast cancer survivors. Based on an ancient Chinese ritual, teams of up to 22 women row a long boat, usually on a river or lake. Dragon boat racing offers women the opportunity to work together to meet a common goal, increase physical fitness and stamina, and provide and receive support from women in a similar situation (Weisenbach & McDonough, 2014). Women training for dragon boat racing are extremely adherent, with a 66% participation rate in training sessions (Courneya, Blanchard, & Laing, 2001); this suggests a commitment to the team and to their own personal goals. Women who participate in this form of exercise report that it provides an opportunity to regain or achieve a sense of control and is a way to overcome the physical challenges after breast cancer treatment (Sabiston, McDonough, & Crocker, 2007). Finally, dragon boat racing has a positive influence on health-related quality of life with improvements seen in physical fitness, endurance, and core, upper, and lower body strength (Ray & Verhoef, 2013). Improvements in self-esteem, body image, self-confidence, and self-acceptance also are reported.

Prostate Cancer

Men with prostate cancer are at risk for poor outcomes due to weight gain from all causes, including being less active after treatment or from medications used to treat their cancer. Weight gain after diagnosis increases the risk of prostate-specific mortality (hazard ratio 1.93, 95% confidence interval [1.18, 3.16]). Men who are obese at diagnosis have a 47% increased risk of overall mortality compared to men of normal weight (Bonn et al., 2014).

The focus of most of the studies on men with prostate cancer is on those prescribed androgen deprivation therapy (ADT) for advanced or recurrent disease. ADT is known to cause a range of metabolic effects including increased total cholesterol, high-density lipoprotein, and triglycerides. This increases risk for cardiovascular disease and cardiac events in men. ADT also increases the risk for development of insulin resistance and diabetes and causes weight gain and alteration in body habitus, with loss of lean muscle mass and an increase in body fat (Choi & Kam, 2015). These changes can occur as early as three months after initiation of treatment and certainly within six months of starting treatment (Boxer, Kenny, Dowsett, & Taxel, 2005; Harrington, Schwenke, Epstein, & Bailey, 2014). ADT increases percentage body fat by an average of 7.7% and decreases lean muscle mass by an average of 2.7%. The longer the duration of treatment, the greater the risk of weight gain and muscle mass loss (Haseen, Murray, Cardwell, O'Sullivan, & Cantwell, 2010). Although most of the studies on exercise in men on ADT have taken place within the context of rehabilitation after side effects occur, it has been suggested that initiating an exercise regimen soon after the start of these therapies may have better outcomes. Studies of this concept are ongoing (Newton et al., 2009, 2012).

Exercise has been shown to improve the side effects of ADT on body mass and muscle loss after as little as 12 weeks (Storer, Miciek, & Travison, 2012). Resistance training using free weights improved physical function and self-reported disability in one trial. Men in the intervention group were compared to a control group who did stretching. The intervention group performed better on all measures (Winters-Stone, Dobek, et al., 2015). A combination of resistance (free weights) and impact (two-footed jumps) training compared to a stretching regimen also had positive outcomes for men on ADT (Winters-Stone, Dieckmann, et al., 2015). After 12 months, the men in the resistance and impact training group had lost total fat and trunk fat. The authors theorized that this also lowered insulin levels. Combining resistance with aerobic exercise has also shown positive results in both preservation of lean body mass and prevention of weight gain in men who started exercising within 10 days of the initiation of ADT (Cormie et al., 2015). A study of endurance training with 12 weeks of stationary bicycle riding three times per week showed a reduction in body weight and fat mass as well as improved insulin sensitivity (Hvid et al., 2013).

When asked, men with prostate cancer on ADT said they were interested and willing to participate in both resistance and aerobic exercise but that they preferred self-paced programs that were flexible, not scheduled ahead of time, and preferably at home (Harrington, Schwenke, & Epstein, 2013). Barriers to engaging in physical activity for men treated with surgery or radiation therapy include pain, incontinence, fatigue, lack of confidence in ability to exercise effectively, and time pressure (Craike, Livingston, & Botti, 2011). Motivators include feeling better, improved self-esteem, coping with stress, and weight control. In this study, 38.9% of men reported exercising at least five times per week and 11.1% were sedentary. Of note is that most of the men did not recall being encouraged to exercise by any of their healthcare providers.

Combining diet and exercise in a six-month intervention trial showed benefits for men on ADT (O'Neill, Haseen, Murray, O'Sullivan, & Cantwell, 2015). Compared to the men in the control group (usual care), the men who participated in the intervention arm lost weight and a percentage of body fat and saw improvements in physical function. The exercise component (30 minutes of vigorous walking five times per week) could be done at home, and the diet followed was the standard healthy eating guideline of the United Kingdom, which includes more than five servings of fruits and vegetables per day, small amounts of fats only, foods low in salt and sugar, and limited alcohol (less than 28 units per week).

A review of diet and exercise interventions for men with prostate cancer treated with any modality suggested that exercise alone does not lead to weight loss and that diet interventions with or without exercise may be the most effective way of losing weight (Mohamad et al., 2015).

Gynecologic Cancer

As discussed in Chapter 2, obesity is a risk factor for endometrial cancer, and many women with gynecologic cancer are obese. Physical activity is recommended for all cancer survivors not only as part of a healthy lifestyle after cancer but also to control weight gain and aid in weight loss. This may be particularly applicable for survivors of gynecologic cancer, where obesity may play a role in disease recurrence. Survivors of gynecologic cancer may be interested in physical activity, but compliance may be low.

Tyrrell, Keats, and Blanchard (2014) asked 239 women about their preferences for physical activity after gynecologic cancer. Although 37% said they were interested in participating in a program of exercise and physical activity, 33% said they were not and 30% said they might be. Ninety-five percent said they preferred walking to other activities, and 68% said that the preferred time to begin a program was three to six months after treatment. Eighty-one percent wanted to exercise at home, and 79% wanted to exercise in the morning. Most (72%) preferred a supervised program and 87% wanted scheduled sessions. However, wanting to participate and actually participating are two different things; in another study, 85% of the survivors said they were interested in participating in an exercise program but only 8% eventually attended (Rossi et al., 2015). Reasons for not attending included inconvenient class times for the program and the study's requirement for the women to get physician clearance to participate.

In a large study of survivors of gynecologic cancer (N = 5,015), 38% reported functional impairment, including 13% who needed equipment to complete their activities of daily living (Nayak et al., 2016). Thirty-three percent reported physical, mental health, and emotional impairment. Less than half of the sample (45%) met the target for physical activity (30 minutes of activity five days per week), while 40% reported being somewhat active.

Outcomes for endometrial cancer survivors are positive when they engage in physical activity. After a six-month home-based exercise program, participants experienced lower resting heart rate, lower systolic blood pressure, better physical functioning, less pain, and increased energy (Basen-Engquist et al., 2014). The mean body mass index for participants was 34.2 kg/m^2. These obese participants had poorer fitness and higher blood pressure at baseline. They also saw less improvement in their fitness than nonobese participants, but they still experienced improvements in quality of life.

Both endometrial and ovarian cancer present unique challenges for survivors in terms of meeting recommendations for physical activity. Women with endometrial cancer may have treatment that predisposes them to the risk of developing lower limb lymphedema, which is a known barrier to physical activity (Hammer, Brown, Segal, Chu, & Schmitz, 2014). In this study, 36% of women surveyed had lower limb lymphedema and 24% reported pain; these were associated with not participating in physical activity. Thirty-eight percent of the sample reported being sedentary, and 62% participated in exercise at least once a week.

Brown, John, Segal, Chu, and Schmitz (2013) found that endometrial cancer survivors who participated in regular physical activity or walking had a lower incidence of lower limb lymphedema (68% risk reduction for physical activity and 81% risk reduction for walking). Because this was a cross-sectional study, however, the authors cautioned that causality cannot be determined.

Women with ovarian cancer may be sicker on diagnosis. In one study of their exercise and physical activity practices, only 19% met the recommended guidelines for 30 minutes of activity five days per week (Mizrahi et al., 2015). Fifty-eight percent of the women in this study reduced the amount of physical activity they engaged in after diagnosis, while 16% increased their activity levels. Barriers to physical activity included fatigue (37.9%), not having exercise as part of their normal precancer routine (34.7%), lack of discipline (32.6%), and procrastination (27.4%). About 25% stated that they lacked interest in exercising, did not enjoy it, and found that exercise was not a priority in their lives. Twenty percent reported pain as a barrier.

When gynecologic cancer survivors do participate in a physical activity program, positive psychological or physical outcomes are reported. In one study of a home-based exercise intervention, participants noted improved mood and distraction from negative thoughts about their cancer. They also reported less fatigue, positive changes in body shape, and improved physical fitness (Donnelly et al., 2013). Women who participated in aerobic exercise (as opposed to strength exercise) experienced fewer negative impacts in a large study of gynecologic cancer survivors (N = 621) (Crawford, Vallance, Holt, & Courneya, 2016). Women reported less negative body changes and self-evaluation, fewer worries about health, and fewer life interferences. The study was designed to investigate the link between physical activity and post-traumatic growth; however, this was not supported, and less negative outcomes were found instead.

Despite what is known about the role of obesity in cancer-related outcomes, gynecologic cancer survivors may not be informed by their healthcare providers about the importance of physical activity in reducing weight and improving multiple domains of physical and psychological functioning. Clark et al. (2016) found that just 37% of women reported being told by their gynecologic oncologist to engage in physical activity; this is about half of the 62% of women who reported that they were given advice about physical activity by their primary care provider. Twenty-nine percent recalled being told about the link between obesity and endometrial cancer. Forty-eight percent increased their physical activity within three months of their diagnosis. This may be an optimal time to encourage lifestyle changes, as the crisis of diagnosis has passed and women have had their surgery.

Colorectal Cancer

A limited number of studies exist on colorectal cancer survivors and their participation in physical activity. However, several studies have looked at these survivors' identified benefits and barriers to exercise. Benefits included improved health and fitness and weight loss. A small number also reported social and psychological benefits, but a reduction in risk of recurrence was rarely mentioned (Fisher et al., 2015). Barriers were commonly reported in this and other studies and included those related to the physical environment; lack of time and support; lack of encouragement from friends, family, and physician; and physical symptoms linked to the disease and treatment such as fatigue, bowel dysfunction, and generally not feeling well (Lynch, Owen, Hawkes, & Aitken, 2010). Age and impaired mobility were barriers reported in one study. Obesity, depression and anxiety, and pain were also cited (Fisher et al., 2015; van Putten et al., 2015).

Survivors may not be aware of the role that physical activity plays in preventing death from colorectal cancer (Karvinen & Vallance, 2015). Although they may know that exercise may support cardiovascular health and daily functioning, the association with colorectal cancer mortality may not be common knowledge for this group as compared to other cancers (e.g., breast). In a large study of colorectal cancer survivors, only 40% of participants knew that regular exercise reduced their risk of recurrence (Speed-Andrews et al., 2014). Improved fitness was identified by 20.2% of participants, 22.8% thought that exercise would improve their physical health, and 25.9% associated exercise with weight loss. When asked what would make exercise fun, 36.5% responded that exercising with others such as family and friends would achieve this. Factors that were seen as barriers included poor health (16.5%), musculoskeletal pain (14.4%), and cancer treatment effects (9.1%). When asked who would be supportive of their participation in regular exercise, 45.7% of survivors said family, 32.3% said their spouse or partner, 25.1% said friends, and 15.8% said their oncology care provider (Speed-Andrews et al., 2014).

Motivation for Physical Activity

Motivation for physical activity may include positive personal factors as well as negative factors. Positive factors include the belief that exercise makes one feel good, contributes to having a healthy body, and maintains health. Those who exercise may report being invigorated by exercise and enjoying the experience of exercise—these can be viewed as intrinsic motivators. Negative factors of exercise are those that avoid bad consequences, such as avoiding ill health and preventing problems and recurrence (Voege, Bower, Stanton, & Ganz, 2015). Breast cancer survivors may be motivated by factors related to the disease itself, such as improved survival in those who exercise and decreased side effects of treatment such as fatigue (Rogers et al., 2004).

Social support plays a role in exercise, too. In a review of the role of social support and physical activity in cancer survivors, Barber (2012) found that the evidence supports the positive role that social support plays in survivors' engagement in physical activity—especially for female survivors. Most of the studies reviewed were in the breast cancer population. The review concluded that multiple levels of social support (partner, family, friends, healthcare providers) increase survivors' participation in exercise as well as frequency. Through companionship, motivation, and health promotion, social support helps cancer survivors (Barber, 2012).

Ryan and Deci's (2000) theory of self-determination provides a detailed description of how motivation may be involved in physical activity. The basic underpinning of this theory is that motivation falls on a continuum from non–self-determined to self-determined. Motivation is regulated by a variety of sources, from nonregulation, to external regulation, to intrinsic (internal) regulation. The processes involved in regulation depend on whether extrinsic or intrinsic forces are at play, and these result in subsequent behaviors.

People who have no motivation tend to not value the behavior, are unable to control their actions, and are generally incompetent at the behavior—in this case, physical activity and exercise.

When people perform activities to receive a reward or to avoid punishment, they are externally regulated; although they may be compliant, they are dependent on others to initiate and maintain the activity. People who use introjected regulation internalize the regulation of the activity. However, they are not fully accepting of the need for it. These people will do the activity to avoid feeling guilty or anxious. They also may feel some degree of self-worth that is conditional on doing the activity.

The next behavior on the continuum is that of identified regulation, where people recognize the importance of the outcome of doing the activity even though they may not enjoy it.

The final behavior is that of intrinsic motivation, where people do the activity because it is enjoyable and because they derive satisfaction from doing it.

To be successful at integrating physical activity in the long term, people need to feel autonomous in their decision to do the activity. This allows the value of physical activity to be integrated into their own values.

To describe these types of motivation in terms of physical activity:

1. People who show **external regulation** will incorporate physical activity when they are forced to and to avoid punishment in the form of negative comments or because they receive some sort of reward from another person who is watching them and ensuring their compliance. We see this in people who exercise because they are either provided some sort of reward (social acceptance or perhaps having their name listed in a public place) or are punished for not complying (they are called out in front of others for not doing their exercise activity).
2. People who show **introjected regulation** comply with physical activity prescription because they feel guilty if they do not do what they have been told to do. The majority of people fall in this category; they do not enjoy exercising but experience feelings of guilt from not exercising.
3. When people include physical activity in their daily life because they know that it is good for them and will make them feel better, they are said to be **identified regulators**. This applies to many people and perhaps to cancer survivors who fear recurrence. They have been told that physical activity can prevent a recurrence of their cancer and participate for that reason only.
4. Finally, people who love to exercise and do it willingly and of their own volition show **intrinsic regulation** and autonomy. People who enjoy physical activity for the way it makes them feel fall into this category.

Motivating Survivors to Incorporate Physical Activity and Exercise in Their Lives

Many of us, patients and healthcare providers alike, do not like to exercise. We see it as something we "have to do" or "should do," and it is more punishment than pleasure. Trying to persuade or encourage patients to do something that they do not want to do can seem like an uphill battle that no one will win. But, as you have read in the pages of this book, exercise has significant benefits for cancer survivors. Ignoring these and not encouraging patients to be more active is not acceptable.

Some survivors have been physically active their whole lives and are frustrated when they cannot exercise at all during or after treatment because of side effects. These patients will be eager to exercise again once they have permission from their oncology care provider or once they feel well enough. They may get frustrated when they cannot do what they did before or find that their level of fitness has slipped due to the enforced break they took during treatment. These patients are easy to motivate—if they need any external motivation at all. They may need to be encouraged to slow down, to be kind to themselves, and cut themselves some slack as their body recovers and their fitness increases over time.

Other survivors may never have exercised in their entire lives or at least not recently or as adults. They may see exercise as a chore and will find every excuse to not incorporate it into their daily lives, despite what they are told by their oncology care provider. This is a major stumbling block to their acceptance that exercise has multiple benefits. Being told what to do takes away autonomy, and adults like to have autonomy over their decisions. In fact, this challenge of personal autonomy can make people dig their heels in and deliberately avoid any and all forms of exercise, even if they do like it just a little bit! If exercise is seen as a chore, something else to be done in a long list of other "to-dos," it is not likely to be done (because who likes to do chores anyway?).

The key to motivating survivors to exercise may be in helping them to internalize their choice to exercise (promoting autonomy), encouraging them to find a form of exercise that they enjoy (personal reward), and helping them to find personal meaning for including exercise in their daily life (e.g., to feel more energized or less fatigued). What we feel in the moment is more important than any rationalization about how beneficial the activity is to us. Therefore, encouraging survivors to pay attention to what they feel during or after exercise (e.g., heightened well-being or a sense of accomplishment) is more effective than providing them with facts and statistics about outcomes such as lowered risk of recurrence. The latter may be perceived as a potential punishment and may cause fear and anxiety rather than a positive feeling that will reinforce positive behavior.

Segar (2015) suggested that the cycle of motivation rests on seeing exercise as a gift and not a chore; this leads to wanting to get active in a way that is pleasurable to the individual, succeeding in meeting one's goals, experiencing the rewards of feeling better physically and mentally, and having renewed energy and perhaps even some fun. These rewards then fuel people's motivation to continue their activity.

Many cancer survivors may think that they cannot or should not exercise. They may have outdated notions of what constitutes exercise (sweating, being out of breath) and may be afraid of exerting themselves or feel unable to do strenuous exercise because of the side effects of treatment or general loss of physical stamina and strength. Segar (2015) pointed out that people do not need to sweat to gain the benefits of exercise, and everyday activities can count toward the daily recommended total of minutes spent in physical activity. Recent research has shown that brief periods of physical activity, as little as 10 minutes or even less interspersed throughout the day, can improve mood (Bossmann, Kanning, Koudela-Hamila, Hey, & Ebner-Priemer, 2013).

The intensity of exercise and the pleasure (or displeasure) that we experience is associated with how we choose to exercise (Ekkekakis, Parfitt, & Petruzzello, 2011). We naturally choose to increase pleasure and avoid displeasure, and our "exercise memory" may be positive or negative based on what we have experienced in the past. If you were forced to participate in physical exercise as a child and the experience was not a good one (remember being chosen last for the baseball team or becoming winded when running around the field and coming in stone-cold last?), the displeasure will remain with you and lower your tolerance (or interest) for rigorous physical activity. The converse is true; if your memories of exercise are positive (being a high school track star or head cheerleader), your interest in intense physical exercise may bring you pleasure. This dictates, in part, how you view exercise as an adult. Some gender differences in exercise intensity exist. Men appear to enjoy higher intensity, and this is associated with reduced physical symptoms. Women prefer less intense activity, and this tends to improve mood more (Asztalos, De Bourdeaudhuij, & Cardon, 2010).

Role of Healthcare Providers

Healthcare providers are seen as being ideally situated to encourage their patients to get physically active because of the trust that patients have in them (Richards, 2015). Some simple ways to increase physical activity in daily life include the following (Segar, 2015):

- Taking the "long cut" (rather than a shortcut) when going about daily activities
- Walking while talking on the phone
- Taking a break from other activities and dancing to a song on the radio, TV, or on a smartphone
- Going for a walk with a partner or spouse, friend, or family member after dinner
- Instead of meeting a friend for coffee in a coffee shop, getting the coffee "to go" and walking around the neighborhood
- Taking one-minute breaks to do some sort of vigorous activity (jumping jacks, lunges, climbing stairs)

These are simple ideas, common sense in many ways, that do not cost money or require special clothes or equipment. They are doable, even for patients undergoing treatment and certainly afterward.

Although rehabilitation programs are being established in greater numbers, frontline healthcare providers play an important role in encouraging patients across the disease trajectory to engage in physical activity to their level of ability. Those who wait until the end of treatment to recommend physical activity to their patients miss the opportunity to increase their patients' well-being and energy and influence other positive outcomes that occur when physical activity is incorporated into the daily lives of patients and their family caregivers.

With increasing specialization in oncology care, it may seem that giving advice about physical activity is the responsibility of an exercise specialist. However, these services are not always available, affordable, or accessible to all patients. Simple commonsense advice about not being sedentary and finding ways to include walking or other forms of physical activity is well within the scope of practice of all oncology care providers. A Cochrane review of interventions to promote regular exercise in cancer survivors concluded that although studies show poor adherence to recommended exercise guidelines, certain actions can be taken to improve this. These include setting program goals, promoting practice and self-monitoring, and encouraging patients to transfer behavior learned in supervised environments to home (Bourke et al., 2013).

CASE VIGNETTE

V.J. is 60 years old and was recently treated for thyroid cancer. She has had some trouble balancing her medications and has gained 20 pounds over the last three months. She reports being depressed, in part because of the weight gain, and is finding it hard to comply with the recommendations of the oncology team to get more active while also watching what she eats. V.J. lives in a retirement complex that has a fully equipped gym, a swimming pool, and walking trails. V.J. says she has no excuses for not exercising but simply does not want to. She finds it frustrating that her nurse keeps telling her to get more exercise.

The SMART acronym can be used to help patients set goals that are specific, measurable, achievable, realistic, and time specific.

Specific Goal

Nurse: I understand that you are unhappy about your recent weight gain and are trying to get rid of those unwanted pounds. You can go about this in a couple of different ways. What is it that YOU want to do?

V.J.: I want to lose this weight as quickly as I can. My niece is getting married in six months, and I want to be thin for her wedding.

Measurable Goal

Nurse: May I suggest that instead of looking at it as 20 pounds that you want to lose, we break it down into smaller chunks? How about we focus on getting rid of five pounds to start? Could we include some walking as part of the plan?

V.J.: I guess I could try to walk a couple of times a week. But I hate going to the gym, so that is not an option!

Achievable Goal

Nurse: I hear you—no gym! If you are willing to incorporate walking, how often do you think you could do that? I want you to succeed, so let's be realistic about what you can do instead of what you should do as a start.

V.J.: Well, I've seen some of the women from the complex walking just after breakfast. If the weather is good, I guess I could join them. I know most of them, and truthfully, they have been nagging me to join them. Maybe I could try for once or twice a week.

Realistic Goal

Nurse: That sounds like an excellent plan, and having company is a big motivator. So, realistically, you could manage once or twice a week to join them? I would suggest that rather than overdoing it once a week, why not join them twice a week, and initially walk with them for 20–30 minutes each time?"

V.J.: I think I could do that. I'm not sure how long they walk for, but they go round and round on the paths in the grounds. I could just stop at 20 minutes if that's what I felt like.

Time-Specific Goal

Nurse: Now, if your niece's wedding is in six months and you want to lose 20 pounds, perhaps we could talk to the nutritionist at the clinic to see what kind of plan she could make for you to help you with losing weight. Six months is a short time, but if you are motivated and keep to your promise of exercising regularly, it may be possible.

Conclusion

Physical activity has the potential to improve physical and psychological outcomes for survivors—and yet, initiating and maintaining recommended weekly targets remains a challenge. Although the increasing evidence supporting the inclusion of physical activity throughout the treatment trajectory and beyond should be motivation enough for survivors, this continues to be a significant challenge for many. However, oncology care providers can be helpful in promoting the benefits of exercise to survivors and motivating them to start and continue with some form of daily physical activity. The following websites contain information on physical activity:

American Cancer Society Guidelines for Nutrition and Physical Activity: www.cancer.org/healthy/eathealthygetactive/acsguidelinesonnutritionphysicalactivityforcancerprevention/acs-guidelines-on-nutrition-and-physical-activity-for-cancer-prevention-guidelines

American College of Sports Medicine: www.acsm.org/about-acsm/media-room/news-releases/2011/08/01/acsm-issues-new-recommendations-on-quantity-and-quality-of-exercise

Every Body Walk!: http://everybodywalk.org

References

Anton, P.M., Partridge, J.A., & Morrissy, M.J. (2013). Cancer caregivers' perceptions of an exercise and nutrition program. *Supportive Care in Cancer, 21,* 803–810. doi:10.1007/s00520-012-1583-8

Asztalos, M., De Bourdeaudhuij, I., & Cardon, G. (2010). The relationship between physical activity and mental health varies across activity intensity levels and dimensions of mental health among women and men. *Public Health Nutrition, 13,* 1207–1214. doi:10.1017/S1368980009992825

Backman, M., Browall, M., Sundberg, C.J., & Wengström, Y. (2015). Experiencing health—Physical activity during adjuvant chemotherapy treatment for women with breast cancer. *European Journal of Oncology Nursing, 21,* 160–167. doi:10.1016/j.ejon.2015.09.007

Balneaves, L.G., Van Patten, C., Truant, T.L., Kelly, M.T., Neil, S.E., & Campbell, K.L. (2014). Breast cancer survivors' perspectives on a weight loss and physical activity lifestyle intervention. *Supportive Care in Cancer, 22,* 2057–2065. doi:10.1007/s00520-014-2185-4

Barber, F.D. (2012). Social support and physical activity engagement by cancer survivors [Online exclusive]. *Clinical Journal of Oncology Nursing, 16,* E84–E98. doi:10.1188/12.CJON.E84-E98

Basen-Engquist, K., Carmack, C., Brown, J., Jhingran, A., Baum, G., Song, J., … Lu, K.H. (2014). Response to an exercise intervention after endometrial cancer: Differences between obese and non-obese survivors. *Gynecologic Oncology, 133,* 48–55. doi:10.1016/j.ygyno.2014.01.025

Bonn, S.E., Wiklund, F., Sjölander, A., Szulkin, R., Stattin, P., Holmberg, E., … Bälter, K. (2014). Body mass index and weight change in men with prostate cancer: Progression and mortality. *Cancer Causes and Control, 25,* 933–943. doi:10.1007/s10552-014-0393-3

Bossmann, T., Kanning, M., Koudela-Hamila, S., Hey, S., & Ebner-Priemer, U.W. (2013). The association between short periods of everyday life activities and affective states: A replication study using ambulatory assessment. *Frontiers in Psychology, 4.* doi:10.3389/fpsyg.2013.00102

Bourke, L., Homer, K.E., Thaha, M.A., Steed, L., Rosario, D.J., Robb, K., … Taylor, S.J.C. (2013). Interventions for promoting habitual exercise in people living with and beyond cancer. *Cochrane Database of Systematic Reviews, 2013*(9). doi:10.1002/14651858.CD010192.pub2

Boxer, R.S., Kenny, A.M., Dowsett, R., & Taxel, P. (2005). The effect of 6 months of androgen deprivation therapy on muscle and fat mass in older men with localized prostate cancer. *Aging Male, 8,* 207–212. doi:10.1080/13685530500361226

Brown, J.C., John, G.M., Segal, S., Chu, C.S., & Schmitz, K.H. (2013). Physical activity and lower limb lymphedema among uterine cancer survivors. *Medical Science in Sports and Exercise, 45,* 2091–2097. doi:10.1249/MSS.0b013e318299afd4

Brunet, J., Burke, S.M., & Sabiston, C.M. (2013). The benefits of being self-determined in promoting physical activity and affective well-being among women recently treated for breast cancer. *Psycho-Oncology, 22,* 2245–2252. doi:10.1002/pon.3287

Bulmer, S.M., Howell, J., Ackerman, L., & Fedric, R. (2012). Women's perceived benefits of exercise during and after breast cancer treatment. *Women and Health, 52,* 771–787. doi:10.1080/03630242.2012.725707

Burke, S.M., & Utley, A. (2013). Psychosocial rehabilitation and recovery: The role of physical activity. *Disability and Rehabilitation, 35,* 2029. doi:10.3109/09638288.2013.824170

Charlier, C., Van Hoof, E., Pauwels, E., Lechner, L., Spittaels, H., Bourgois, J., & De Bourdeaudhuij, I. (2012). Treatment-related and psychosocial variables in explaining physical activity in women three weeks to six months post-treatment of breast cancer. *Patient Education and Counseling, 89,* 171–177. doi:10.1016/j.pec.2012.06.029

Choi, S.M., & Kam, S.C. (2015). Metabolic effects of androgen deprivation therapy. *Korean Journal of Urology, 56,* 12–18. doi:10.4111/kju.2015.56.1.12

Clark, L.H., Ko, E.M., Kernodle, A., Harris, A., Moore, D.T., Gehrig, P.A., & Bae-Jump, V. (2016). Endometrial cancer survivors' perceptions of provider obesity counseling and attempted behavior change: Are we seizing the moment? *International Journal of Gynecological Cancer, 26,* 318–324. doi:10.1097/IGC.0000000000000596

Cormie, P., Galvão, D.A., Spry, N., Joseph, D., Chee, R., Taaffe, D.R., … Newton, R.U. (2015). Can supervised exercise prevent treatment toxicity in patients with prostate cancer initiating androgen-deprivation therapy: A randomised controlled trial. *BJU International, 115*, 256–266. doi:10.1111/bju.12646

Courneya, K.S., Blanchard, C.M., & Laing, D.M. (2001). Exercise adherence in breast cancer survivors training for a dragon boat race competition: A preliminary investigation. *Psycho-Oncology, 10*, 444–452. doi:10.1002/pon.524

Craike, M.J., Livingston, P.M., & Botti, M. (2011). An exploratory study of the factors that influence physical activity for prostate cancer survivors. *Supportive Care in Cancer, 19*, 1019–1028. doi:10.1007/s00520-010-0929-3

Crawford, J.J., Vallance, J.K., Holt, N.L., & Courneya, K.S. (2016). Extreme sport/adventure activity correlates in gynecologic cancer survivors. *American Journal of Health Behavior, 40*, 172–181. doi:10.5993/AJHB.40.2.2

Demark-Wahnefried, W., Rogers, L.Q., Alfano, C.M., Thomson, C.A., Courneya, K.S., Meyerhardt, J.A., … Ligibel, J.A. (2015). Practical clinical interventions for diet, physical activity, and weight control in cancer survivors. *CA: A Cancer Journal for Clinicians, 65*, 167–189. doi:10.3322/caac.21265

Djuric, Z., Ellsworth, J.S., Weldon, A.L., Ren, J., Richardson, C.R., Resnicow, K., … Sen, A. (2011). A diet and exercise intervention during chemotherapy for breast cancer. *Open Obesity Journal, 3*, 87–97. doi:10.2174/1876823701103010087

Donnelly, C.M., Lowe-Strong, A., Rankin, J.P., Campbell, A., Blaney, J.M., & Gracey, J.H. (2013). A focus group study exploring gynecological cancer survivors' experiences and perceptions of participating in a RCT testing the efficacy of a home-based physical activity intervention. *Supportive Care in Cancer, 21*, 1697–1708. doi:10.1007/s00520-012-1716-0

Ekkekakis, P., Parfitt, G., & Petruzzello, S. (2011). The pleasure and displeasure people feel when they exercise at different intensities. *Sports Medicine, 41*, 641–671. doi:10.2165/11590680-000000000-00000

Fisher, A., Wardle, J., Beeken, R.J., Croker, H., Williams, K., & Grimmett, C. (2015). Perceived barriers and benefits to physical activity in colorectal cancer patients. *Supportive Care in Cancer, 24*, 903–910. doi:10.1007/s00520-015-2860-0

Fong, D.Y., Ho, J.W., Hui, B.P., Lee, A.M., Macfarlane, D.J., Leung, S.S., … Cheng, K.K. (2012). Physical activity for cancer survivors: Meta-analysis of randomised controlled trials. *BMJ, 344*, e70. doi:10.1136/bmj.e70

Forsythe, L.P., Alfano, C.M., George, S.M., McTiernan, A., Baumgartner, K.B., Bernstein, L., & Ballard-Barbash, R. (2013). Pain in long-term breast cancer survivors: The role of body mass index, physical activity, and sedentary behavior. *Breast Cancer Research and Treatment, 137*, 617–630. doi:10.1007/s10549-012-2335-7

Foucaut, A.M., Berthouze-Aranda, S.E., Touillaud, M., Kempf-Lépine, A.S., Baudinet, C., Meyrand, R., … Fervers, B. (2014). Reduction of health risk factors through an adapted physical activity program in patients with breast cancer. *Supportive Care in Cancer, 22*, 1097–1104. doi:10.1007/s00520-013-2065-3

Greenlee, H.A., Crew, K.D., Mata, J.M., McKinley, P.S., Rundle, A.G., Zhang, W., … Hershman, D.L. (2013). A pilot randomized controlled trial of a commercial diet and exercise weight loss program in minority breast cancer survivors. *Obesity, 21*, 65–76. doi:10.1002/oby.20245

Hammer, S.M., Brown, J.C., Segal, S., Chu, C.S., & Schmitz, K.H. (2014). Cancer-related impairments influence physical activity in uterine cancer survivors. *Medical Science in Sports and Exercise, 46*, 2195–2201. doi:10.1249/MSS.0000000000000360

Harrington, J.M., Schwenke, D.C., & Epstein, D.R. (2013). Exercise preferences among men with prostate cancer receiving androgen-deprivation therapy [Online exclusive]. *Oncology Nursing Forum, 40*, E358–E367. doi:10.1188/13.ONF.E358-E367

Harrington, J.M., Schwenke, D.C., Epstein, D.R., & Bailey, D.E., Jr. (2014). Androgen-deprivation therapy and metabolic syndrome in men with prostate cancer. *Oncology Nursing Forum, 41*, 21–29. doi:10.1188/14.ONF.21-29

Haseen, F., Murray, L.J., Cardwell, C.R., O'Sullivan, J.M., & Cantwell, M.M. (2010). The effect of androgen deprivation therapy on body composition in men with prostate cancer: Systematic review and meta-analysis. *Journal of Cancer Survivorship, 4,* 128–139. doi:10.1007/s11764-009-0114-1

Hojan, K., Molińska-Glura, M., & Milecki, P. (2013). Physical activity and body composition, body physique, and quality of life in premenopausal breast cancer patients during endocrine therapy—A feasibility study. *Acta Oncologica, 5,* 319–326. doi:10.3109/0284186X.2012.744468

Hvid, T., Winding, K., Rinnov, A., Dejgaard, T., Thomsen, C., Iversen, P., ... Pedersen, B.K. (2013). Endurance training improves insulin sensitivity and body composition in prostate cancer patients treated with androgen deprivation therapy. *Endocrine-Related Cancer, 20,* 621–632. doi:10.1530/ERC-12-0393

Karvinen, K., & Vallance, J. (2015). Breast and colon cancer survivors' expectations about physical activity for improving survival. *Oncology Nursing Forum, 42,* 527–533. doi:10.1188/15.ONF.527-533

Kim, J.J., Shin, Y.A., & Suk, M.H. (2015). Effect of a 12-week walking exercise program on body composition and immune cell count in patients with breast cancer who are undergoing chemotherapy. *Journal of Exercise Nutrition and Biochemistry, 19,* 255–262. doi:10.5717/jenb.2015.15092812

Knobf, M.T., Insogna, K., DiPietro, L., Fennie, C., & Thompson, A.S. (2008). An aerobic weight-loaded pilot exercise intervention for breast cancer survivors: Bone remodeling and body composition outcomes. *Biologic Research for Nursing, 10,* 34–43. doi:10.1177/1099800408320579

Loh, S.Y., Chew, S.L., & Lee, S.Y. (2011). Physical activity and women with breast cancer: Insights from expert patients. *Asian Pacific Journal of Cancer Prevention, 12,* 87–94.

Loprinzi, P.D., & Cardinal, B.J. (2012). Effects of physical activity on common side effects of breast cancer treatment. *Breast Cancer, 19,* 4–10. doi:10.1007/s12282-011-0292-3

Lynch, B.M., Owen, N., Hawkes, A.L., & Aitken, J.F. (2010). Perceived barriers to physical activity for colorectal cancer survivors. *Supportive Care in Cancer, 18,* 729–734. doi:10.1007/s00520-009-0705-4

Maley, M., Warren, B.S., & Devine, C.M. (2013). A second chance: Meanings of body weight, diet, and physical activity to women who have experienced cancer. *Journal of Nutrition Education and Behavior, 45,* 232–239. doi:10.1016/j.jneb.2012.10.009

Mizrahi, D., Naumann, F., Broderick, C., Samara, J., Ryan, M., & Friedlander, M. (2015). Quantifying physical activity and the associated barriers for women with ovarian cancer. *International Journal of Gynecological Cancer, 25,* 577–583. doi:10.1097/IGC.0000000000000349

Mohamad, H., McNeill, G., Haseen, F., N'Dow, J., Craig, L.C., & Heys, S.D. (2015). The effect of dietary and exercise interventions on body weight in prostate cancer patients: A systematic review. *Nutrition and Cancer, 67,* 43–60. doi:10.1080/01635581.2015.976313

Mohammadi, S., Sulaiman, S., Koon, P.B., Amani, R., & Hosseini, S.M. (2013). Impact of healthy eating practices and physical activity on quality of life among breast cancer survivors. *Asian Pacific Journal of Cancer Prevention, 14,* 481–487. doi:10.7314/APJCP.2013.14.1.481

Nayak, P., Vernon, S.W., Savas, L.S., Basen-Engquist, K., Morgan, R.O., & Elting, L.S. (2016). Functional impairment and physical activity adherence among gynecologic cancer survivors: A population-based study. *International Journal of Gynecologic Cancer, 26,* 381–388. doi:10.1097/IGC.0000000000000620

Newton, R.U., Taaffe, D.R., Spry, N., Cormie, P., Chambers, S.K., Gardiner, R.A., ... Galvão, D.A. (2012). Can exercise ameliorate treatment toxicity during the initial phase of testosterone deprivation in prostate cancer patients? Is this more effective than delayed rehabilitation? *BMC Cancer, 12,* 432. doi:10.1186/1471-2407-12-432

Newton, R.U., Taaffe, D.R., Spry, N., Gardiner, R.A., Levin, G., Wall, B., ... Galvão, D.A. (2009). A phase III clinical trial of exercise modalities on treatment side-effects in men receiving therapy for prostate cancer. *BMC Cancer, 9,* 210. doi:10.1186/1471-2407-9-210

Nock, N.L., Owusu, C., Flocke, S., Krejci, S.A., Kullman, E.L., Austin, K., ... Berger, N.A. (2015). A community-based exercise and support group program improves quality of life in African-American breast cancer survivors: A quantitative and qualitative analysis. *International Journal of Sports and Exercise Medicine, 1*(3).

O'Neill, R.F., Haseen, F., Murray, L.J., O'Sullivan, J.M., & Cantwell, M.M. (2015). A randomised controlled trial to evaluate the efficacy of a 6–month dietary and physical activity intervention for patients receiving androgen deprivation therapy for prostate cancer. *Journal of Cancer Survivorship, 9,* 431–440. doi:10.1007/s11764-014-0417-8

Paxton, R.J., Phillips, K.L., Jones, L.A., Chang, S., Taylor, W.C., Courneya, K.S., & Pierce, J.P. (2012). Associations among physical activity, body mass index, and health-related quality of life by race/ethnicity in a diverse sample of breast cancer survivors. *Cancer, 118,* 4024–4031. doi:10.1002/cncr.27389

Ray, H.A., & Verhoef, M.J. (2013). Dragon boat racing and health-related quality of life of breast cancer survivors: A mixed methods evaluation. *BMC Complementary and Alternative Medicine, 13,* 205. doi:10.1186/1472-6882-13-205

Richards, E. (2015). The evolution of physical activity promotion. *American Journal of Nursing, 115*(8), 50–54. doi:10.1097/01.NAJ.0000470400.28683.97

Rock, C.L., Flatt, S.W., Byers, T.E., Colditz, G.A., Demark-Wahnefried, W., Ganz, P.A., ... Wyatt, H. (2015). Results of the Exercise and Nutrition to Enhance Recovery and Good Health for You (ENERGY) Trial: A behavioral weight loss intervention in overweight or obese breast cancer survivors. *Journal of Clinical Oncology, 33,* 3169–3176. doi:10.1200/JCO.2015.61.1095

Rogers, L.Q., Matevey, C., Hopkins-Price, P., Shah, P., Dunnington, G., & Courneya, K.S. (2004). Exploring social cognitive theory constructs for promoting exercise among breast cancer patients. *Cancer Nursing, 27,* 462–473.

Rossi, A., Moadel-Robblee, A., Garber, C.E., Kuo, D., Goldberg, G., Einstein, M., & Nevadunsky, N. (2015). Physical activity for an ethnically diverse sample of endometrial cancer survivors: A needs assessment and pilot intervention. *Journal of Gynecologic Oncology, 26,* 141–147. doi:10.3802/jgo.2015.26.2.141

Ryan, R., & Deci, E. (2000). Self-determination theory and the facilitation of intrinsic motivation, social development, and well-being. *American Psychologist, 55,* 68–78. doi:10.1037/0003-066X.55.1.68

Sabiston, C.M., McDonough, M.H., & Crocker, P.R. (2007). Psychosocial experiences of breast cancer survivors involved in a dragon boat program: Exploring links to positive psychological growth. *Journal of Sport and Exercise Psychology, 29,* 419–438. doi:10.1123/jsep.29.4.419

Schmitz, K., Courneya, K., Matthews, C., Demark-Wahnefried, W., Galvão, D., Pinto, B., ... Schwartz, A. (2010). American College of Sports Medicine roundtable on exercise guidelines for cancer survivors. *Medicine and Science in Sports and Exercise, 42,* 1409–1426. doi:10.1249/MSS.0b013e3181e0c112

Scott, E., Daley, A.J., Doll, H., Woodroofe, N., Coleman, R.E., Mutrie, N., ... Saxton, J.M. (2013). Effects of an exercise and hypocaloric healthy eating program on biomarkers associated with long-term prognosis after early-stage breast cancer: A randomized controlled trial. *Cancer Causes and Control, 24,* 181–191. doi:10.1007/s10552-012-0104-x

Segar, M. (2015). *No sweat: How the simple science of motivation can bring you a lifetime of fitness.* New York, NY: AMACOM.

Sheppard, V.B., Hicks, J., Makambi, K., Hurtado-de-Mendoza, A., Demark-Wahnefried, W., & Adams-Campbell, L. (2016). The feasibility and acceptability of a diet and exercise trial in overweight and obese black breast cancer survivors: The Stepping STONE study. *Contemporary Clinical Trials, 46,* 106–113. doi:10.1016/j.cct.2015.12.005

Speed-Andrews, A.E., McGowan, E.L., Rhodes, R., Blanchard, C., Culos-Reed, S., Friedenreich, C., & Courneya, K. (2014). Identification and evaluation of the salient physical activity beliefs of colorectal cancer survivors. *Cancer Nursing, 37,* 14–22. doi:10.1097/NCC.0b013e3182813972

Storer, T.W., Miciek, R., & Travison, T.G. (2012). Muscle function, physical performance and body composition changes in men with prostate cancer undergoing androgen deprivation therapy. *Asian Journal of Andrology, 14,* 204–221. doi:10.1038/aja.2011.104

Swisher, A.K., Abraham, J., Bonner, D., Gilleland, D., Hobbs, G., Kurian, S., ... Vona-Davis, L. (2015). Exercise and dietary advice intervention for survivors of triple-negative breast cancer: Effects on body fat, physical function, quality of life, and adipokine profile. *Supportive Care in Cancer, 23,* 2995–3003. doi:10.1007/s00520-015-2667-z

Travier, N., Fonseca-Nunes, A., Javierre, C., Guillamo, E., Arribas, L., Peiró, I., ... Agudo, A. (2014). Effect of a diet and physical activity intervention on body weight and nutritional patterns in overweight and obese breast cancer survivors. *Medical Oncology, 31,* 783. doi:10.1007/s12032-013-0783-5

Tyrrell, A., Keats, M., & Blanchard, C. (2014). The physical activity preferences of gynecologic cancer survivors. *Oncology Nursing Forum, 41,* 461–469. doi:10.1188/14.ONF.461-469

U.S. Department of Health and Human Services. (2008). 2008 physical activity guidelines for Americans. Retrieved from https://health.gov/paguidelines/pdf/paguide.pdf

van Putten, M., Husson, O., Mols, F., Luyer, M.D., van de Poll-Franse, L.V., & Ezendam, N.P. (2015). Correlates of physical activity among colorectal cancer survivors: Results from the longitudinal population-based profiles registry. *Supportive Care in Cancer, 24,* 573–583. doi:10.1007/s00520-015-2816-4

Voege, P., Bower, J.E., Stanton, A.L., & Ganz, P. (2015). Motivations associated with physical activity in young breast cancer survivors. *Psychology, Health and Medicine, 20,* 393–399. doi:10.1080/13548506.2014.955033

Voskuil, D.W., van Nes, J.G., Junggeburt, J.M., van de Velde, C.J., van Leeuwen, F.E., & de Haes, J.C. (2010). Maintenance of physical activity and body weight in relation to subsequent quality of life in postmenopausal breast cancer patients. *Annals of Oncology, 21,* 2094–2101. doi:10.1093/annonc/mdq151

Weisenbach, B.B., & McDonough, M.H. (2014). Breast cancer survivors' decisions to join a dragon boating team. *Journal of Sport and Exercise Psychology, 36,* 564–573. doi:10.1123/jsep.2014-0037

Whitehead, S., & Lavelle, K. (2009). Older breast cancer survivors' views and preferences for physical activity. *Qualitative Health Research, 19,* 894–906. doi:10.1177/1049732309337523

Winters-Stone, K.M., Dieckmann, N., Maddalozzo, G.F., Bennett, J.A., Ryan, C.W., & Beer, T.M. (2015). Resistance exercise reduces body fat and insulin during androgen-deprivation therapy for prostate cancer. *Oncology Nursing Forum, 42,* 348–356. doi:10.1188/15.ONF.348-356

Winters-Stone, K.M., Dobek, J.C., Bennett, J.A., Dieckmann, N.F., Maddalozzo, G.F., Ryan, C.W., & Beer, T.M. (2015). Resistance training reduces disability in prostate cancer survivors on androgen deprivation therapy: Evidence from a randomized controlled trial. *Archives of Physical Medicine and Rehabilitation, 96,* 7–14. doi:10.1016/j.apmr.2014.08.010

Winters-Stone, K.M., Dobek, J.C., Nail, L., Bennett, J.A., Leo, M.C., Naik, A., & Schwartz, A. (2011). Strength training stops bone loss and builds muscle in postmenopausal breast cancer survivors: A randomized, controlled trial. *Breast Cancer Research and Treatment, 127,* 447–456. doi:10.1007/s10549-011-1444-z

Young, A., Weltzien, E., Kwan, M., Castillo, A., Caan, B., & Kroenke, C.H. (2014). Pre- to post-diagnosis weight change and associations with physical functional limitations in breast cancer survivors. *Journal of Cancer Survivorship, 8,* 539–547. doi:10.1007/s11764-014-0356-4

Chapter 6

Barriers and Facilitators to Lifestyle Change

It is well accepted that losing weight or maintaining a healthy weight and getting regular exercise has a host of health benefits for adults and especially cancer survivors. However, making changes to one's lifestyle is challenging at the best of times, and encouraging patients to do this at a difficult time in their lives may prove to be almost impossible. This chapter describes the evidence associated with lifestyle changes for cancer survivors. An emphasis is placed on breast, prostate, and colorectal cancers because this is where the majority of the research focuses. Much of the research describes the barriers and facilitators to lifestyle change as identified by cancer survivors and their oncology team members.

Physical Activity

Breast Cancer

Although breast cancer survivors recognize the importance of physical activity during and after treatment, just over half (56%) of women reported regularly exercising after treatment (Demark-Wahnefried, Peterson, McBride, Lipkus, & Clipp, 2000). Women may acknowledge that exercise improves general health, prevents disease recurrence, and improves physical appearance (Sander, Wilson, Izzo, Mountford, & Hayes, 2012), but significant barriers to regular participation still exist. Some of these are disease related, such as postsurgical pain, lymphedema, fatigue, neuropathy, and joint pain from adjuvant endocrine therapy (Sander et al., 2012). Other barriers include bad weather, lack of access to a gym or equipment, no one to exercise with, and time constraints related to employment or family responsibilities (Brunet, Burke, & Sabiston, 2013). In another study, 52% of breast cancer survivors said they were too busy to exercise, and

51% said they had no willpower (Ottenbacher et al., 2011). African American women identified obesity as a barrier to participating in exercise, as well as lack of energy, self-discipline, and interest (Oyekanmi & Paxton, 2014). For women undergoing chemotherapy, significant barriers to exercise include nausea, fatigue, and feeling unwell (Courneya et al., 2008). Barriers still exist five years after treatment for many women. Barriers include lack of motivation, dislike of the gym, weight gain, and caregiving and family responsibilities. Older age and comorbidities are also cited as barriers (Hefferon, Murphy, McLeod, Mutrie, & Campbell, 2013).

Australian researchers concluded that perceived barriers to exercise outweigh perceived benefits (Gho, Munro, Jones, & Steele, 2014). In this study, breast cancer survivors stated that benefits to exercise included improvements in physical health and functioning and feelings of well-being. Other benefits included social contact, improvements in job performance, increase in muscle strength, and weight loss. Despite more than 60% of participants citing these benefits, the negative aspects or barriers resulted in fewer of the women in the study being sufficiently active.

One study identified some interesting factors that influenced the women not to exercise (Sander et al., 2012). In the study, some women reported that their friends and family encouraged them to rest and to avoid household tasks. Fear and confusion about the relationship between exercise and the development of lymphedema was also noted. The women reported that lack of accurate information about the association of exercise and lymphedema and what constituted safe exercise was a barrier. Conflicting information that they found on the Internet contributed to their confusion, fear, and avoidance of exercise.

Prostate Cancer

Although physical activity is part of many men's daily routines, treatment for prostate cancer can affect their ability or motivation to exercise. In one study, 62% of prostate cancer survivors exercised routinely (Demark-Wahnefried et al., 2000). Motivators of physical activity include psychological benefits such as feeling better, experiencing relaxation and reduction of stress, and maintaining a positive outlook about the cancer diagnosis. Physical benefits include weight management, increased energy, and positive self-esteem. Social motivators include opportunities to spend time with family, friends, and partners while exercising. Barriers include lack of time, comorbidities, older age and physical decline, and not having confidence in the ability to exercise following treatment (Craike, Livingston, & Botti, 2011). In addition, Ottenbacher et al. (2011) found that 44% of the men they surveyed said that they had no willpower and that bad weather posed a barrier to exercise. In men treated with androgen deprivation therapy, fatigue and lack of motivation were barriers to physical activity, while physician and spousal encouragement were facilitators (Keogh, Patel, MacLeod, & Masters, 2014).

Healthy Eating and Weight Loss

Breast Cancer

In a large study including both breast and prostate cancer survivors, 47% of women ate more than five servings of fruits and vegetables a day, and 73% restricted their fat intake to less than 30% of total intake, thus complying with general recommendations (Demark-Wahnefried et al., 2000).

Barriers to healthy eating for women with breast cancer include temptation at the holidays and on special occasions, not being able to control impulses to eat whatever they want, and preferring the taste of high-fat foods (Ventura et al., 2013). In addition, eating out a lot and being from a cultural group whose traditions include high-fat foods also account for challenges to healthy eating.

Prostate Cancer

As with other cancers, the diagnosis of prostate cancer provides an impetus for dietary and physical activity change. In one study, 58% of newly diagnosed men made changes to the way they eat, predominantly by including more fruits and vegetables and less fat in their diet (Satia, Walsh, & Pruthi, 2009). Demark-Wahnefried et al. (2000) assessed intake of fruits, vegetables, and fat in a sample of men with prostate cancer. Sixty-two percent of the men consumed fewer than five servings of fruits and vegetables per day, and 75% of these men were not planning on increasing their intake. Thirty percent of these men had dietary fat intake greater than 30%, and 83% were not planning on changing this.

A diagnosis of cancer often precipitates the inclusion of physical activity in the life of men with prostate cancer. Satia et al. (2009) reported that 67% of the men interviewed in their study exercised regularly before diagnosis, and this increased to 75% after diagnosis. Facilitators included physician recommendation and family support. Barriers included lack of time and treatment-related factors such as incontinence.

In another study, 40% of the participants were on active surveillance. The men reported being uncertain about the link between diet and cancer; however, 59% of the total sample reported changing their diet (Avery et al., 2014). They most often included more tomatoes or tomato products in their diet, but they also increased their intake of fruits and vegetables and decreased fat consumption. The reasons they gave for these changes were to maintain their health, to be fit for when they had treatment, to prevent progression or recurrence, to prevent other cancers, and to feel like they were "doing something," particularly if they were following an active surveillance protocol. Men who had surgery or radiation reported that they thought that dietary changes were not necessary, as they viewed themselves as being cured of cancer.

In contrast, Coa, Smith, Klassen, Thorpe, and Caulfield (2015) found that men did not make dietary changes after diagnosis but did say they were interested in losing weight. Barriers to healthy eating included lack of willpower and preference for high-fat foods to healthier alternatives, not having the necessary self-discipline to make dietary changes, lack of time to prepare healthy foods, and lack of access to healthy foods while at work. These men relied heavily on their spouse or partner to purchase and prepare their meals, and some men blamed their spouse for their poor eating habits.

Colorectal Cancer

Eating a healthy diet and getting regular exercise is important for colorectal cancer survivors as well. When surveyed about their knowledge of and adherence to dietary guidelines, 72% of colorectal cancer survivors chose lean meats and poultry as well as low- or nonfat dairy and beans as part of their diet. There was resistance to this, however; 26% said that eating a healthy diet took too much effort. Participants who were female and had more education were more aware of the recommendations to avoid processed meats, saturated fats, and trans fats (Hawkins, Berkowitz, & Rodriguez, 2015).

Barriers to regular physical exercise in this population are similar to other cancers and include fatigue, impaired mobility, age, chemotherapy side effects, pain, loss of appetite and weight loss, depression, and obesity (Fisher et al., 2015; van Putten et al., 2015). Regarding oneself as already active enough and lack of encouragement from family and friends have also been reported (Lynch, Owen, Hawkes, & Aitken, 2010), as well as fear of leakage from a stoma for those with an ostomy.

Facilitators of physical activity in colorectal cancer survivors include improved physical health and fitness and weight loss (Fisher et al., 2015). In this study, the association with a reduction in the risk of recurrence was not cited.

Role of Healthcare Providers

Whether or not cancer survivors incorporate lifestyle changes is in part motivated by internal factors. (See Chapter 7 for a discussion on stages of change.) However, the concept of cancer as a "teachable moment" (Demark-Wahnefried, Aziz, Rowland, & Pinto, 2005) is widely accepted as a time when lifestyle change may be accepted by patients and their families (Husebø, Dyrstad, Søreide, & Bru, 2013). Many physicians in general do not actively promote healthier lifestyles to their patients, regardless of whether the patient is a cancer survivor or a healthy adult (Smith et al., 2011). In a study of a nationally representative sample of primary care providers, less than half reported giving specific lifestyle advice to adult patients and were more likely to talk about physical activity than diet and weight control. It can be challenging to talk about diet. Healthcare providers recognize that many overweight and obese patients have tried and failed to lose weight, and this undermines their confidence that they can be successful if they try again (Phillips et al., 2012).

Despite increasing evidence of the association between lifestyle and cancer recurrence, not all oncology care providers agree that the time to encourage lifestyle change is at or near diagnosis. Coa et al. (2015) interviewed oncologists and primary care providers for their views on this. Disagreement was noted among those interviewed about when is the best time for a "teachable moment." Some thought that talking about dietary changes should happen soon after diagnosis so that patients could make changes as needed to eat a healthy diet during treatment and prevent weight gain. Others felt that waiting until after treatment was preferred, as the treatment regimen itself is a challenge for patients; however, they also felt that there was a narrow window of opportunity after treatment, when patients would be motivated to make changes in their diet. Others agreed with this and raised the issue of weight loss during chemotherapy and the need for most patients to consume sufficient calories at this time. All those interviewed stressed that patients need to hear messages about healthy eating and dietary change repeatedly over the course of treatment so that they hear the message when they are ready to make changes; the timing is not going to be the same for all patients. Participants in the study also stated that those patients at high risk for recurrence may be more motivated to make changes, as diet is something that they can have control over in an essentially uncontrollable situation. Young patients were thought to be more motivated to make changes, as they are seen to be more concerned about their mortality than older patients. Fatigue was seen as a major barrier to making dietary changes, as it limited patients' energy to access and prepare healthy foods. In addition, oncologists said they would talk to patients about dietary change only if they had strong evidence on which to base their recommendations. Primary care providers saw this as something that needed to be discussed with all patients.

In another report from the same group, Baker et al. (2015) described the practices of the same oncology care providers concerning weight management in their patients. Many of those interviewed stated that they discussed weight management with their patients; however, some said that this was not their clinical responsibility or that time constraints prevented them from having the discussion. For those who did talk to their patients, starting the conversation during treatment was seen as appropriate because it gave control to their patients and empowered them to make changes at a time when they did not have much power. The discussion is usually framed within the clinical role of the care provider. For example, a surgeon will discuss weight in the context of preparing for surgery, or a nurse may talk about it in the context of survivorship and reducing the risk of recurrence. The issue of unintentional weight loss was mentioned by some of the participants who felt that this was the focus of many patients during treatment who were scared of losing weight; however, they did state that some patients were more worried about weight gain as a side effect of treatment.

The oncology care providers also gave information about weight management and physical activity in different ways. Some provided patients with pamphlets and videos after assessing each patient's behaviors at the time and whether they were ready to make lifestyle changes. Others referred patients to a nutritionist or trainer or told their patients to search the Internet for advice. For those who counseled their patients about lifestyle change, this was often seen as futile and hopeless. Participants recognized personal, social, and environmental challenges faced by their patients, as well as issues with institutional resources and payment barriers.

Gynecologic oncologists recognize the importance of counseling about weight management with their patients. Ninety-five percent of those surveyed said counseling was important, and 82% thought that it would not harm the physician–patient relationship (Jernigan, Tergas, Satin, & Fader, 2013). Those younger than age 42 were more likely to report receiving education about weight management for patients, and 81.5% said that they referred patients to bariatric specialists, primary care providers, or commercial weight-loss programs. Fifty-four percent addressed healthy eating with their patients on a regular basis and 61.6% discussed physical activity, but less than a third (29.1%) discussed goal weight with patients.

In a review of strategies that oncology care providers can use to assist patients with lifestyle change, the following facts are described (Demark Wahnefried et al., 2015):

1. The oncology care provider is a trusted and valued professional who has significant influence with patients as well as repeated interactions over the course of active treatment and beyond.
2. Primary care providers are important partners, as weight management and activity counseling is a routine part of the care they provide to patients.
3. Weight management and exercise specialists can provide the intensive support that many patients require.
4. A number of organizations and associations exist that can be useful to oncology care providers for information and referrals (see Table 6-1).
5. Many cancer survivors may benefit from commercial weight management and exercise programs, particularly once they are no longer in active treatment.

Table 6-1. Resources for Cancer Survivors and the Oncology Care Community to Promote Weight Management, Physical Activity, and a Healthy Diet*

Domain	Resource
Weight management	Academy of Nutrition and Dietetics: Board-Certified Specialists in Oncology Nutrition https://ams.eatright.org/eweb/DynamicPage.aspx?Site=CDRNEW&WebKey=8EADAFE4-F1E1-4309-B21C-66D3CC2AA112
	American Cancer Society (library of brochures and web-based information for cancer survivors) www.cancer.org/treatment/survivorshipduringandaftertreatment/index
	American Institute for Cancer Research (library of brochures and web-based information for cancer survivors) www.aicr.org/patients-survivors
	American Society of Clinical Oncology (oncologist and patient guides) www.asco.org/practice-guidelines/cancer-care-initiatives/prevention-survivorship/obesity-cancer
	Livestrong (web-based diet and exercise information and calorie tracker) www.livestrong.com

(Continued on next page)

Table 6-1. Resources for Cancer Survivors and the Oncology Care Community to Promote Weight Management, Physical Activity, and a Healthy Diet* *(Continued)*

Domain	Resource
Physical activity	American Cancer Society (library of brochures and web-based information for cancer survivors) www.cancer.org/treatment/survivorshipduringandaftertreatment/index
	American College of Sports Medicine: Exercise is Medicine Campaign http://exerciseismedicine.org
	American Institute for Cancer Research (library of brochures and web-based information for cancer survivors) www.aicr.org/patients-survivors
	Livestrong (web-based exercise information) www.livestrong.com
	Livestrong at the YMCA (12-week exercise program) www.livestrong.org/what-we-do/program/livestrong-at-the-ymca
	American College of Sports Medicine (Cancer Exercise Trainer certification) http://certification.acsm.org/acsm-cancer-exercise-trainer
	Silver Sneakers www.silversneakers.com
Healthy diet	Academy of Nutrition and Dietetics: Board-Certified Specialists in Oncology Nutrition https://ams.eatright.org/eweb/DynamicPage.aspx?Site=CDRNEW&WebKey=8EADAFE4-F1E1-4309-B21C-66D3CC2AA112
	American Cancer Society (library of brochures and web-based information for cancer survivors) www.cancer.org/treatment/survivorshipduringandaftertreatment/index
	American Institute for Cancer Research (library of brochures and web-based information for cancer survivors) www.aicr.org/patients-survivors

* Programs that are for profit or those that are only available regionally are not included.

Note. From "Practical Clinical Interventions for Diet, Physical Activity, and Weight Control in Cancer Survivors," by W. Demark-Wahnefried, L.Q. Rogers, C.M. Alfano, C.A. Thomson, K.S. Courneya, J.A. Meyerhardt, … J.A. Ligibel, 2015, *CA: A Cancer Journal for Clinicians, 65,* p. 183. Copyright 2015 by American Cancer Society. Reprinted with permission.

CASE VIGNETTE

B.W. completed multimodality treatment for colorectal cancer just over three months ago and has an ileostomy that he hopes will be reversed in the upcoming months. He has always been heavyset and is now on the cusp of being clinically obese. As a younger man, he was an enthusiastic baseball player, but the increasing demands of running his own courier service in the small town where he lives and now his cancer diagnosis have resulted in him getting no exercise at all.

On his most recent visit for follow-up care, B.W. is shocked when the nurse tells him he has gained almost 10 pounds since his last visit. His wife, S.W., is with him, and she shakes her head when he tells the nurse that he had no idea how he could have gained that much weight.

"The only exercise you get is going to the fridge to get a beer or to the pantry to get another handful of potato chips!" she tells him.

"What are you talking about?" replies B.W., his voice raised enough that other patients in the waiting room look up to see what is going on. "It's not MY fault! It's all that food you keep shoving at me!"

Questions

1. How can the nurse deal with the immediate situation, which looks like it might escalate into a verbal argument?
2. How can the nurse help this couple to see how they both can participate in solving B.W.'s weight gain problem?

SPIKES Model

Using the SPIKES model (Setting, Perception, Invitation, Knowledge, Empathy, and Summary and Strategy), the nurse can help B.W. and his wife identify where changes can be made (Kaplan, 2010). (The SPIKES model is discussed in more depth in Chapter 7.)

Setting

Nurse: Why don't we carry on this conversation in the examination room where I have some resources that I can share with you?

Perception

Nurse: So, B.W. and S.W., have you noticed a change in how and what you are eating as a couple? S.W., you seem to have one idea, but B.W. seems to think something different.

S.W.: Well, to be honest, he did lose some weight when he was having the chemo, but I was scared that he was losing too much weight, so I started baking more and buying more snacks.

B.W.: She's a fine baker. And it's not like I've held back on snacking since the end of my treatment either, so it's not all her fault.

Invitation

Nurse: Can we talk about what you both can do to eat healthier now that treatment is over?

S.W.: I know what to do, but I don't know if he wants to do what's necessary.

B.W.: Give the nurse a chance. I know that I need to lose some of this weight. I'm not feeling that great with this big tummy of mine.

Knowledge

Nurse: Many family members are afraid that their loved one will lose weight, so they make changes to their usual diet to prevent that. Then it's hard to go back to the old way, or they just get used to eating differently. You can do a couple of common-sense things, like serving smaller portions, eating fewer baked goods—no matter how great they taste—and, of course, getting more exercise.

B.W.: You're not going to insist that I go to the gym, are you?

Empathy

Nurse: You don't have to do anything you don't want to do. I understand that this might feel like yet another thing you have to do, and I know you are tired of treatment and so many visits to the cancer center.

B.W.: I've read that getting exercise can help patients feel better and less tired, but that doesn't make much sense to me.

S.W.: To me as well. Won't it make him even more tired?

Nurse: I know it sounds strange, but the research does show that exercise reduces fatigue for cancer survivors, especially for people who have had radiation therapy. You don't have to make any decisions today; I just wanted to plant a seed. We can talk more at your next appointment.

Summary and Strategy

Nurse: So, let's recap. S.W., you are going to think about not tempting him with your baking. B.W., you are going to think about perhaps including some sort of physical exercise in your day. Does that sound right to you?

B.W.: You're putting words in my mouth, nurse, but yes, I will think about it—and who knows? I may even try to do something about getting rid of this extra baggage I'm carrying around by my next appointment.

Conclusion

As many of us know from personal experience, making lifestyle changes is difficult for some and nearly impossible for others. If it were easy, as the saying goes, we would

ALL eat healthy foods and exercise regularly. But it is not easy; making changes to diet and physical activity is difficult and requires not only willpower and self-discipline but support, guidance, and knowledge of valid interventions. A range of resources can assist oncology care providers in guiding and encouraging their patients to make these lifestyle changes. However, to understand why patients sometimes fail to make recommended changes, it is important to recognize that adherence to recommendations is limited.

References

Avery, K.N., Donovan, J.L., Horwood, J., Neal, D.E., Hamdy, F.C., Parker, C., ... Lane, A. (2014). The importance of dietary change for men diagnosed with and at risk of prostate cancer: A multicentre interview study with men, their partners and health professionals. *BMC Family Practice, 15,* 81. doi:10.1186/1471-2296-15-81

Baker, A.M., Smith, K.C., Coa, K.I., Helzlsouer, K.J., Caulfield, L.E., Peairs, K.S., ... Klassen, A.C. (2015). Clinical care providers' perspectives on body size and weight management among long-term cancer survivors. *Integrative Cancer Therapy, 14,* 240–248. doi:10.1177/1534735415572882

Brunet, J., Burke, S.M., & Sabiston, C.M. (2013). The benefits of being self-determined in promoting physical activity and affective well-being among women recently treated for breast cancer. *Psycho-Oncology, 22,* 2245–2252. doi:10.1002/pon.3287

Coa, K.I., Smith, K.C., Klassen, A.C., Thorpe, R.J., Jr., & Caulfield, L.E. (2015). Exploring important influences on the healthfulness of prostate cancer survivors' diets. *Qualitative Health Research, 25,* 857–870. doi:10.1177/1049732315580108

Courneya, K.S., McKenzie, D.C., Reid, R.D., Mackey, J.R., Gelmon, K., Friedenreich, C.M., ... Segal, R.J. (2008). Barriers to supervised exercise training in a randomized controlled trial of breast cancer patients receiving chemotherapy. *Annals of Behavioral Medicine, 35,* 116–122. doi:10.1007/s12160-007-9009-4

Craike, M.J., Livingston, P.M., & Botti, M. (2011). An exploratory study of the factors that influence physical activity for prostate cancer survivors. *Supportive Care in Cancer, 19,* 1019–1028. doi:10.1007/s00520-010-0929-3

Demark-Wahnefried, W., Aziz, N.M., Rowland, J.H., & Pinto, B.M. (2005). Riding the crest of the teachable moment: Promoting long-term health after the diagnosis of cancer. *Journal of Clinical Oncology, 23,* 5814–5830. doi:10.1200/JCO.2005.01.230

Demark-Wahnefried, W., Peterson, B., McBride, C., Lipkus, I., & Clipp, E. (2000). Current health behaviors and readiness to pursue life-style changes among men and women diagnosed with early stage prostate and breast carcinomas. *Cancer, 88,* 674–684. doi:10.1002/(SICI)1097-0142(20000201)88:3<674::AID-CNCR26>3.0.CO;2-R

Demark-Wahnefried, W., Rogers, L.Q., Alfano, C.M., Thomson, C.A., Courneya, K.S., Meyerhardt, J.A., ... Ligibel, J.A. (2015). Practical clinical interventions for diet, physical activity, and weight control in cancer survivors. *CA: A Cancer Journal for Clinicians, 65,* 167–189. doi:10.3322/caac.21265

Fisher, A., Wardle, J., Beeken, R.J., Croker, H., Williams, K., & Grimmett, C. (2015). Perceived barriers and benefits to physical activity in colorectal cancer patients. *Supportive Care in Cancer, 24,* 903–910. doi:10.1007/s00520-015-2860-0

Gho, S.A., Munro, B.J., Jones, S.C., & Steele, J.R. (2014). Perceived exercise barriers explain exercise participation in Australian women treated for breast cancer better than perceived exercise benefits. *Physical Therapy, 94,* 1765–1774. doi:10.2522/ptj.20130473

Hawkins, N.A., Berkowitz, Z., & Rodriguez, J.L. (2015). Awareness of dietary and alcohol guidelines among colorectal cancer survivors. *American Journal of Preventive Medicine, 49*(Suppl. 5), S509–S517. doi:10.1016/j.amepre.2015.08.012

Hefferon, K., Murphy, H., McLeod, J., Mutrie, N., & Campbell, A. (2013). Understanding barriers to exercise implementation 5-year post-breast cancer diagnosis: A large-scale qualitative study. *Health Education Research, 28,* 843–856. doi:10.1093/her/cyt083

Husebø, A.M.L., Dyrstad, S.M., Søreide, J.A., & Bru, E. (2013). Predicting exercise adherence in cancer patients and survivors: A systematic review and meta-analysis of motivational and behavioural factors. *Journal of Clinical Nursing, 22,* 4–21. doi:10.1111/j.1365-2702.2012.04322.x

Jernigan, A.M., Tergas, A.I., Satin, A.J., & Fader, A.N. (2013). Obesity management in gynecologic cancer survivors: Provider practices and attitudes. *American Journal of Obstetrics and Gynecology, 208,* 408.e1–408.e8. doi:10.1016/j.ajog.2013.02.002

Kaplan, M. (2010). SPIKES: A framework for breaking bad news to patients with cancer. *Clinical Journal of Oncology Nursing, 14,* 514–516. doi:10.1188/10.CJON.514-516

Keogh, J.W., Patel, A., MacLeod, R.D., & Masters, J. (2014). Perceived barriers and facilitators to physical activity in men with prostate cancer: Possible influence of androgen deprivation therapy. *European Journal of Cancer Care, 23,* 263–273. doi:10.1111/ecc.12141

Lynch, B.M., Owen, N., Hawkes, A.L., & Aitken, J.F. (2010). Perceived barriers to physical activity for colorectal cancer survivors. *Supportive Care in Cancer, 18,* 729–734. doi:10.1007/s00520-009-0705-4

Ottenbacher, A.J., Day, R.S., Taylor, W.C., Sharma, S.V., Sloane, R., Snyder, D.C., … Demark-Wahnefried, W. (2011). Exercise among breast and prostate cancer survivors—What are their barriers? *Journal of Cancer Survivorship, 5,* 413–419. doi:10.1007/s11764-011-0184-8

Oyekanmi, G., & Paxton, R.J. (2014). Barriers to physical activity among African American breast cancer survivors. *Psycho-Oncology, 23,* 1314–1317. doi:10.1002/pon.3527

Phillips, K., Wood, F., Spanou, C., Kinnersley, P., Simpson, S.A., & Butler, C.C. (2012). Counselling patients about behaviour change: The challenge of talking about diet. *British Journal of General Practice, 62,* e13–e21. doi:10.3399/bjgp12X616328

Sander, A.P., Wilson, J., Izzo, N., Mountford, S.A., & Hayes, K.W. (2012). Factors that affect decisions about physical activity and exercise in survivors of breast cancer: A qualitative study. *Physical Therapy, 92,* 525–536. doi:10.2522/ptj.20110115

Satia, J.A., Walsh, J.F., & Pruthi, R.S. (2009). Health behavior changes in white and African American prostate cancer survivors. *Cancer Nursing, 32,* 107–117. doi:10.1097/NCC.0b013e3181982d4c

Smith, A.W., Borowski, L.A., Liu, B., Galuska, D.A., Signore, C., Klabunde, C., … Ballard-Barbash, R. (2011). U.S. primary care physicians' diet, physical activity, and weight-related care of adult patients. *American Journal of Preventive Medicine, 41,* 33–42. doi:10.1016/j.amepre.2011.03.017

van Putten, M., Husson, O., Mols, F., Luyer, M.D., van de Poll-Franse, L.V., & Ezendam, N.P. (2015). Correlates of physical activity among colorectal cancer survivors: Results from the longitudinal population-based profiles registry. *Supportive Care in Cancer, 24,* 573–583. doi:10.1007/s00520-015-2816-4

Ventura, E.E., Ganz, P.A., Bower, J.E., Abascal, L., Petersen, L., Stanton, A.L., & Crespi, C.M. (2013). Barriers to physical activity and healthy eating in young breast cancer survivors: Modifiable risk factors and associations with body mass index. *Breast Cancer Research and Treatment, 142,* 423–433. doi:10.1007/s10549-013-2749-x

Chapter 7
Communicating About Weight Issues With Patients

Oncology care providers have many challenging conversations with patients and their families. From delivering the initial diagnosis of cancer to discussing end-of-life options, difficult conversations are commonplace and something we are educated to do. Over the past decades, we have seen many taboo topics come into the open. Talking about death and dying was once taboo. Discussing sexuality and sexual health with cancer survivors was widely neglected. Many of us find it daunting to talk about overweight and obesity with our patients; this is the latest "elephant in the room" in oncology.

Much of what we know about communication on this topic comes from primary care. The U.S. Preventive Services Task Force (USPSTF) published a statement in 2012 that recommended screening all adults for obesity. Screening was given a grade B recommendation, indicating a high certainty that the net benefit to the individual is moderate or moderate certainty that the benefit is moderate to substantial. The recommendation is that clinicians should offer or refer patients with a body mass index (BMI) of 30 kg/m^2 or higher to intensive, multicomponent behavioral interventions to help them reduce their body mass. The statement includes recognition of the role of obesity in the development of multiple conditions, including certain types of cancer (liver, kidney, breast, endometrial, prostate, and colon) (USPSTF, 2012).

Many of our patients with cancer are overweight or even obese when diagnosed with cancer, and their family members are, too. A significant number of our patients gain weight during and after their chemotherapy or endocrine treatments. We see our patients over the course of these treatments and for years afterward. So, why is it so difficult to talk about this? This chapter will describe the challenges we have in discussing this topic with our patients (and among ourselves). It will provide the reader with a toolkit of resources to initiate the conversation and to offer assistance to patients. It also will address the sensitive issue of personal weight in healthcare providers and how it may affect our willingness or refusal to talk about this topic with our patients.

Language

What words do we use when talking about overweight and obesity? Body mass or weight is associated with negative feelings, and the language we use in the clinical setting can influence how our advice is received. If we want patients to understand the importance of managing their weight, we need to get the message across in a way that is acceptable to them and that will not create offense or misunderstanding. Healthcare providers may prefer to use medical terms when describing the need to lose weight, while patients may prefer plain language descriptors. Healthcare providers tend to use less sensitive phrases such as "You need to be healthy" rather than "You need to lose weight," believing that it will make patients feel less anxious (Gudzune, Clark, Appel, & Bennett, 2012).

The public has a preference for the language used by healthcare providers. Puhl, Peterson, and Luedicke (2013) reported that the general public prefers the terms *weight* and *unhealthy weight*. The terms regarded as most motivating to lose weight are *unhealthy weight* and *overweight*. In this study, 19% of respondents said that they would avoid future interactions with a healthcare provider and 21% said they would seek a new healthcare provider if they felt stigmatized by the provider about their weight.

What is the difference in word choice, and where is the common ground for patients and providers? Tailor and Ogden (2009) explored this issue in their study with primary care providers and patients who rated their preferences for certain words. The study found that physicians did not want to use the word *obese* with their patients and preferred to talk in euphemisms such as "Your weight may be damaging to your health" (47% preferred this term). Alternatives were "You are overweight" (21%) and "You need to lose some weight" (16%).

When patients were presented with these options, being told "You are obese" resulted in feeling that the problem was serious and had greater emotional impact than the euphemism that the physicians preferred. However, if the patient was not obese, the term *obese* was associated with feelings of anxiety and depression. Obese patients reported the opposite; for them, the euphemism "Your weight may be damaging to your health" was associated with depression and anxiety.

In this study, using plain language was indicative of the seriousness of the problem and may have been the trigger for behavior change, particularly among those who were obese. In another study, people who were seeking help in losing weight were asked to rate 12 terms in order of acceptability (Dutton et al., 2010). Their physicians were also asked to rate these terms based on how likely they were to use the terms in the clinical setting. The patients, all of whom were obese, rated the terms as presented alongside physician preference in Table 7-1. Although the patients and physicians agreed about some preferred terms (*weight* being preferred by both patients and physicians) and nonpreferred terms (*fatness* and *excess fat* being the least acceptable), a range of terms exist in common usage that would be problematic for patients if their healthcare provider used them.

This topic is an emotional one for many, and using a term that elicits strong emotions is not conducive to patient acceptance of advice about managing weight (see Table 7-1).

Table 7-1. Patient and Provider Preferences* for Language to Describe Overweight and Obesity

Patients	Physicians
Weight	Weight
Body mass index (BMI)	Excess weight
Unhealthy body weight	Unhealthy body weight
Unhealthy BMI	BMI
Weight problem	Weight problem
Excess weight	Unhealthy BMI
Overweight status	Overweight status
Heaviness	Obesity
Obesity	Large size
Large size	Heaviness
Excess fat	Excess fat
Fatness	Fatness

* Language is listed from most to least acceptable. White shading indicates negative opinion.

Note. Based on information from Dutton et al., 2010.

Discussing Weight Loss

Initiating a conversation about weight, no matter how difficult, is an important first step in helping patients understand the health effects of being overweight or obese and then planning to do something to change this. When healthcare providers tell their patients that they are overweight or obese, it is more likely to result in the patients understanding that their weight affects their health. In one study, this message resulted in those patients who were told that their weight was negatively affecting their health being nine times more aware of this than those who were not told (Durant, Bartman, Person, Collins, & Austin, 2009). Overweight and obese individuals recognized that they had a weight problem if their physician told them so. They also were more likely to have made an attempt to lose weight in the previous 12 months. But only 45.2% of overweight and 66.4% of obese individuals reported being told that they were overweight or obese (Post et al., 2011). Nurses believe that counseling about healthy lifestyles is within their scope of practice but are more likely to encourage increasing physical activity (44% of respondents) than reducing caloric intake (25%) (Kable et al., 2015).

When healthcare providers tell overweight or obese patients that they need to lose weight, the patients are more likely to do so. Pool et al. (2014) reported that patients were twice as likely to lose 5% of their body mass if told by their physician that they needed to lose weight. Female physicians are more likely to tell their patients that they need to lose weight and refer patients for weight-loss counseling (Dutton et al., 2014). However, healthcare providers and patients may not agree on just how overweight the patient is. When patients think that their healthcare provider is judging them based on their weight, they are almost five times more likely to try to lose weight (odds ratio [OR] 4.96; 95% confidence interval [CI] [1.96, 11.14]). However, they may be more successful at actually losing weight if the discussion does not make them feel judged (Gudzune, Beach, Roter, & Cooper, 2013).

Physicians tend to see their patients as more overweight and with greater potential for negative health effects than their patients do. Patients, especially women, believe that they will be more successful at losing weight than their physicians think they will be (Befort et al., 2006). This creates the potential for challenging conversations about the need to lose weight and patients' ability to do so. If patients perceive that their healthcare provider has a negative perception about their motivation and ability to lose weight, they may avoid talking about it or ignore what they are being told. In turn, healthcare providers may find it frustrating to counsel patients who seem unrealistic about their situation.

Barriers to providing advice about weight management occur in three areas: the patient, the healthcare provider, and the healthcare environment. Patient barriers include lack of motivation, stigma and denial, previous experience (success or failure) of weight loss, and cost of services such as weight-loss groups. Practitioner barriers include lack of skill and time, the high levels of effort needed to motivate patients and monitor their efforts, and lack of support for practitioners to manage overweight and obese patients (Sinfield, Baker, Pollard, & Tang, 2013).

It has been suggested that a diagnosis of cancer provides a "teachable moment" for many individuals and their family members (Coa, Smith, Klassen, Thorpe, & Caulfield, 2015). When someone is newly diagnosed with cancer, circumstances exist that create an impetus for behavior change; this reflects some of the basic tenets of the Health Belief Model (Lawson & Flocke, 2009). The diagnosis itself is a cue to action; cancer is universally perceived as a significant threat to health and life itself; and patients may sincerely want to do something that will help themselves in the situation.

In a review of lifestyle changes after a cancer diagnosis, it was concluded that cancer survivors do initiate changes in diet (Demark-Wahnefried, Aziz, Rowland,

& Pinto, 2005). However, less than 50% of survivors maintain this lifestyle change. The authors reported that 70% of breast and prostate cancer survivors are overweight or obese after treatment. Barriers to making dietary changes include food preferences, lack of knowledge about what constitutes a healthy diet, difficulty breaking lifelong eating habits, lack of progress leading to giving up, food as a solace and coping mechanism, and lack of support from social networks who may hold differing views on weight in the context of cancer (Coa et al., 2015). Although friends and family may make changes to their own diet in response to a cancer diagnosis in someone they know or love, this is not universal and not as common as one might predict. In one study among friends and family members, 58.5% increased their intake of fruit and vegetables, 53.2% decreased their intake of fat, 52.8% increased their fiber intake, and 50.4% decreased their consumption of fast food (Humpel, Magee, & Jones, 2007). This compares to over 80% of individuals with cancer changing their dietary intake.

Healthcare providers may be more likely to include guidance about weight management when there is strong evidence to support it, but when and how to do this remains challenging. The authors suggested introducing the topic early in the treatment period so that those who want to make changes will be encouraged to do so (Coa et al., 2015). Repeated messaging about the role of diet and exercise along the treatment trajectory and during survivorship care will remind those who have not initiated changes that this is important to prevent recurrence and the development of comorbidities.

Motivation to Change

The Transtheoretical Model, developed by James Prochaska and Carlo DiClemente, is a widely used model that describes the stages that individuals move through when attempting behavior change. One stage precedes the other, and, although patients may remain in one stage longer or shorter than in others, they have to move through each stage before proceeding to the next. They may experience regression or repetition of certain stages, depending on the abilities or circumstances of the individual. The model has five stages: precontemplation, contemplation, preparation, action, and, finally, maintenance of the changes achieved (www.prochange.com/transtheoretical-model-of-behavior-change).

The *precontemplation* stage is when the individual is not ready to make any changes. This may result from lack of information about how the behavior may affect health or may reflect avoidance or denial that the behavior or situation is potentially or actually harmful to the individual's health.

The *contemplation* stage is when the individual is getting ready to make a change (typically within six months following the precontemplation phase, according to this model). In this stage, people usually weigh the pros and cons of making the change. This can result in ambivalence and inertia that may last for a long time.

A state of readiness to change is the hallmark of the *preparation* stage. In this stage, the individual has a plan that he or she intends to follow and the intention to activate the plan in the immediate future.

The *action* stage is said to occur when changes have occurred in the past six months and the individual is actively engaged in doing things differently. This is usually followed by the *maintenance* stage, when confidence in the ability to continue with the changes made is high and the individual tries to prevent a relapse to the old behavior.

It is important to be aware of these stages of change because they reflect how likely it is that the patient is able to do what we suggest to change his or her lifestyle. Trying to move patients to make changes when they do not fully understand what they need to do and why (as in the precontemplation stage) will result in frustration for the healthcare provider and conflict with patients. Some patients may be in a stage of readiness for far longer than we think is necessary, and they will not be willing or able to move into the action stage and make the changes until they are ready.

Models to Assist in Talking to Patients

A number of models are used in practice to initiate conversation about weight management and lifestyle change with patients. Although none of these are specific to the topic, some have been used successfully with other kinds of behavior modification or when addressing sensitive topics.

5 A's Model

This model has been used successfully in tobacco cessation for years and is thought to be appropriate for other lifestyle modifications, including healthy eating and physical exercise prescription. This model consists of five activities that the healthcare provider is encouraged to use with patients to increase motivation and maximize success: ask, advise, assess, assist, and arrange. Examples of the stages with descriptions and appropriate questions or statements are presented in Table 7-2.

This method of counseling patients to make lifestyle changes has been associated with success. In a study of physician communication with patients who were overweight and obese, physicians used one of the "A's" in 83% of encounters. To avoid bias, both physicians and patients were told that the study was about preventive health, not weight loss (Alexander et al., 2011). Patients were most often asked about weight loss (77%) and advised to lose weight (68%). The least frequent activity was assessment (4%), but patients were assisted 13% of the time, and follow-up was arranged 5% of the time. When patients were given direct advice or were assessed by the physician, they were more likely to report confidence in their ability to lose weight. Those patients who had follow-up arranged by the physician also were more likely to have lost weight.

Table 7-2. 5 A's Model

Action	Definition	Example
Ask	Healthcare provider asks patients about their weight, eating habits, etc.	"How concerned are you about your weight?" "What do you think are the reasons you have gained weight during treatment?"
Advise	Healthcare provider gives patients clear and direct information	"Getting 30 minutes of exercise per day will help you lose weight." "Your weight may raise the risk of your cancer coming back."
Assess	Healthcare provider assesses patients' willingness to make changes	"Do you see yourself doing something about your weight gain in the near future?"
Assist	Healthcare provider counsels patients and provides self-help material	"How do you feel about being able to make some changes in your daily diet?"
Arrange	Healthcare provider arranges for follow-up or for referral to nutritionist	"I'd like to see you again in two weeks to see if you have lost any weight." "We have a nutritionist on staff who can help you with meal planning."

Note. Based on information from Jay et al., 2010.

Jay, Gillespie, Schlair, Sherman, and Kalet (2010) studied physician communication with obese patients and found that although 85% of the patients received some counseling about weight management, physicians did not use the full 5 A's of the model. Most of the patient-reported activities focused on assessing rather than on assisting or arranging. Those patients who stated that they were highly motivated to lose weight reported that they received more counseling techniques based on the 5 A's model. This may reflect greater interest on the part of the patient, which resulted in greater engagement on the part of the physician. With each additional counseling technique that was added, a 30% increase was noted in the odds of patient motivation (OR 1.31; 95% CI [1.11, 1.55]) through better eating (OR 1.23; 95% CI [1.06, 1.44]) or getting more exercise (OR 1.14; 95% CI [1.00, 1.31]). If the physician was perceived to be more patient centered, the odds of intention to eat better improved almost three times (OR 2.96; 95% CI [1.10, 8.47]).

Of note is that the Centers for Medicare and Medicaid Services requires the use of the 5 A's technique when providing counseling for obese patients (Gudzune et al., 2012).

Ask-Tell-Ask Model

This simple three-step model uses a straightforward approach in which the healthcare provider *asks* permission of the patient to provide information, then *tells* the patient what he or she wants to know, and then once again *asks* if further clarification is needed or wanted (Svarovsky, 2013).

The Brief Negotiation Interview

Chapter 4 introduced the concept of motivational interviewing, a widely accepted method of facilitating behavior change such as initiating and maintaining a healthy lifestyle (see also Chapter 8). A modification of this, the Brief Negotiation Interview (BNI), has been suggested as a facilitator of decision making in health care (Pantalon et al., 2013) and may be useful as a framework for discussions about managing weight with overweight and obese patients. This four-step process may be used as presented; however, the authors suggested that using even just one of the steps may be sufficient in motivating patients to make a decision about changing aspects of their lifestyle.

Step 1: Ask the Patient's Permission to Discuss the Topic and Reinforce Patient Autonomy

By asking permission, and then abiding by the patient's decision to discuss weight or strategies to manage weight, the healthcare provider is showing respect for the patient and also supporting patient autonomy in deciding whether to address his or her weight at this time. A statement such as, "Are you interested in talking about some changes you might be willing to make in order to lose the weight you have gained during treatment? I have some suggestions for you but it is up to you if you want to talk about this or not" seeks permission as well as promotes patient autonomy.

Step 2: Provide Feedback of the Patient's Response to the Information Provided

This step involves active listening on the part of the healthcare provider and then reflecting back to the patient what was said. This provides an opportunity for the healthcare provider to highlight anything that the patient has said that may indicate a willingness to change. An example of an opening for this step could be, "It sounds as though you are experiencing significant fatigue as you recover from your chemotherapy treatment. But at the same time, you seem to be interested in doing whatever you can to return to your usual activities. Do you want to talk about that a little more?"

Step 3: Enhance Motivation With One or More of the Following Strategies

By focusing on patient indicators of willingness to change behavior, the healthcare provider has the opportunity to reinforce motivation. This can be accomplished by any one of the following suggestions:

- Ask the patient, "Why change?" Eliciting the patient's reasons for making changes provides further opportunities to reinforce this motivation and captures personally relevant factors that can be emphasized to further empower and motivate the patient.
- Assess motivation by asking the patient, "On a scale of 1 to 10, how ready are you to make a change in the way you eat?" After the patient responds, and if applicable, ask, "Why didn't you pick a number less than a 4?" This allows the patient a chance to respond in a positive way, suggesting facilitators for behavior change rather than negative reasons.
- Repeatedly ask and talk about motivation rather than resistance. Questions such as, "What would it mean to you if you could find a way to visit the farmers' market every week rather than relying on take-out food for dinner every night?" prompt constructive responses rather than negative ones.

Step 4: Ask the Patient What the Next Step Is

By asking the patient about his or her readiness or willingness, the healthcare provider reinforces patient autonomy and control rather than compliance with any suggestions. A question such as, "What, if any, next step are you willing to make?" puts the patient in control. Adding "if any" in the question encourages the patient to think of the decision as one that he or she is making, and, as a result, the patient is more likely to carry through.

SPIKES Model

The SPIKES model was originally developed to discuss distressing topics with patients (Kaplan, 2010). The acronym SPIKES stands for Setting, Perception, Invitation, Knowledge, Empathy, and Summary and Strategy. This six-step process can be used to initiate a discussion about lifestyle change or weight management but is less patient centered than other models.

Setting—Choose a setting that is private and where disturbances are minimized, as would be ideal for any discussion where the content is potentially sensitive or likely to evoke an emotional response. Avoid distractions and focus on the patient in a calm and engaged manner.

Perception—Seek out the patient's understanding of the situation or the topic to be discussed. Unlike other models that follow a more permissive pattern (such as BNI or motivational interviewing), this model suggests that the healthcare provider directly asks the patient what he or she understands about the topic and its importance. This allows for assessment of the patient's knowledge or understanding of the situation and can form a baseline for the discussion to follow.

Invitation—Ask the patient how much (or how little) he or she wants to know and what kind of information might be useful.

Knowledge—Present information about behavior change or weight management to the patient based on his or her level of interest or understanding. Medical jargon and terminology is to be avoided, and clear, direct statements should be used. It also is important to repeatedly check that the patient understands what is being told.

Empathy—Convey empathy by acknowledging the emotions and reactions of the patient in response to the information.

Summary and Strategy—In this final stage, summarize the information given to the patient, provide the next steps, and ask if clarification is needed.

NURSE Framework

Another framework for discussing sensitive topics is NURSE. This acronym stands for the responses that healthcare providers can use when responding to emotional cues from patients when discussing topics that are upsetting or sensitive. Much like the SPIKES framework, it is fairly directive and provider centered. At the same time, it encourages patients to express their feelings.

Naming—This involves the healthcare provider naming the emotion that the patient appears to be experiencing. For example, if the healthcare provider asks the patient, "I wonder if you're angry with me for bringing up the topic of your weight," this allows the patient to own and express any emotions so that they are out in the open.

Understanding—This allows for an exploration of the emotion the patient is feeling and for the healthcare provider to validate that feeling. For example, "What your anger is telling me is that you are not comfortable talking about your weight or that you don't want to talk at the present time. Please clarify this for me."

Respecting—Communication that indicates to the patient that he or she is respected as an individual with his or her own thoughts and feelings is important in building a therapeutic relationship. For example, "I understand that this is a topic that you don't want to talk about. However, it is important for your health, and I hope that you will think about this and we can have a conversation about it at some other time."

Supporting—Communication showing that the healthcare provider supports the patient's decision and will provide any resources necessary to make the behavior change when the patient is ready is vital to the patient–provider relationship. For example, "Although you may not be ready to talk about this now, here is my phone number, as well as a list of resources, that you can use at any time in the future. Your decision to not talk about this today will not influence the care you receive in any way."

Exploring—In this final stage, the healthcare provider asks direct questions for clarification and understanding, thus allowing the patient to express any emotions more fully and openly. For example, "What else would you like to tell me about what you are thinking or feeling about our talk today?"

The Overweight and Obese Healthcare Provider

One of the barriers to addressing weight issues in patients is the personal weight status of the healthcare provider. If a nurse, physician, or allied health provider is overweight or obese, do they feel comfortable talking to patients about their weight status and recommending that they lose weight? Given the ubiquity of overweight and obesity in North American society, it is reasonable to assume that some of those individuals are healthcare providers. A study of 760 RNs found that 54% of those surveyed reported being overweight or obese with a mean BMI of 27.2 kg/m^2 (Miller, Alpert, & Cross, 2008).

So, how does this affect patient–provider interactions, particularly in the area of weight management strategies? Although evidence is mixed with suggestions of weight bias on the part of patients, evidence of acceptance of overweight healthcare providers also exists. Hash, Munna, Vogel, and Bason (2003) found that patients were more likely to be receptive to health advice from nonobese physicians. A study investigated public perception of normal-weight, overweight, and obese physicians (Puhl, Gold, Luedicke, & DePierre, 2013). The study found that respondents were more mistrustful of overweight and obese physicians and were less likely to follow their instructions. These biases were present even if the respondents themselves were overweight or obese. Conversely, overweight and obese patients were found to trust diet advice from overweight or obese healthcare providers compared to providers who were of normal weight (Bleich, Gudzune, Bennett, Jarlenski, & Cooper, 2013). Overweight healthcare providers may be seen by their patients as more empathetic. For patients who were lacking in motivation, healthcare providers with similar weight issues were preferred (Leske, Strodl, & Hou, 2012).

Physician weight affects the care they provide, with overweight or obese physicians less likely to talk about weight loss than their colleagues with normal BMIs (18% vs. 30%) and less confident in their ability to provide weight management advice (37% vs. 53%). When physicians thought that a patient's BMI was the same or higher than their own, they were more likely to initiate a discussion about weight (Bleich, Bennett, Gudzune, & Cooper, 2012).

What does this mean for overweight or obese healthcare providers? Is this a rationale for not talking about weight with patients who are overweight or obese themselves? Given the evidence that overweight and obesity influences the development and recurrence of cancer, it would be irresponsible to ignore this evidence and not raise the topic with patients. Our own weight issues can provide a bridge to empathy and understanding, as suggested by the participants in Leske's (2012) study, where the healthcare providers' own struggles were seen in a positive light. Overweight nurses in one study reported that they were conscious of their size and felt guilty about how they were perceived by patients as potential role models (Brown & Thompson, 2007). Although some of the nurses used their own weight status as a source of empathy, they also made assumptions about overweight patients and based their advice on personal beliefs rather than evidence. They also tended to be more critical of obese patients in part because of their own self-criticism.

Patients may be more accepting of advice from someone who has "been there, done that" rather than from someone who appears to have never had to deal with the challenges of being overweight or obese. Although everyone has the right to withhold personal information, and some healthcare providers may believe that it is wrong to share one's own personal life and health issues with patients, it is not difficult for patients to be able to judge for themselves whether we could stand to lose a pound or ten! Pretending that your own weight is invisible creates another elephant in the room, and it might be better to address that quickly and efficiently and then move on to evidence-based and not personally biased information to guide patients.

The following is an example of a conversation using the 5 A's model that an overweight healthcare provider might have with a patient.

Ask

Provider: In the three months since we last saw you, you've gained five pounds. What do you think is going on, and is this something you want to talk about?

Patient: Yeah, I noticed that my pants are tight around my middle. I've always had a weight issue, and I read in the pamphlet they gave me at the drugstore that those pills I'm taking cause weight gain. But what am I supposed to do?

Advise

Provider: You are correct. The pills you are taking to prevent a recurrence of your cancer are known to increase your risk of gaining weight. But this is something that you can be proactive about.

Patient: I have to tell you, this is just one more thing to deal with, and I'm pretty much at the end of my rope. It's been a rough year for me and my family, and I'm not sure that I can deal with having to lose weight on top of everything else.

Assess

Provider: It sounds like you're feeling overwhelmed. Given that your weight is something you've dealt with in the past, do you feel OK about managing the five pounds you've gained in the past couple of months, or would you like some help with that? I've been dealing with weight issues my whole life, too. Five pounds can become 10 and then 20 pretty quickly, and that's a whole different challenge.

Patient: Oh, so maybe you understand how hard this is. I know about that slippery slope and how if I'm not watching myself, my weight can get completely out of control. I know in my head what I have to do, but I'm really tired, and I just want to feel normal again. Having to think about dieting makes me feel like I have to do something else that I don't want to do. I didn't want to do the chemo and I had to. Now, I have to take these pills that are going to make me gain even more. I just want to give up right now!

Assist

Provider: I understand how frustrating this feels. And it also sounds like you feel you have no control. I have some information you might find helpful, and we also have a nutritionist and exercise specialist who we can refer you to.

Patient: I don't know . . . frankly, the fewer times I have to come back here, the better. But I do want to do something about this. I really don't want to have to buy a new wardrobe in a bigger size.

Arrange

Provider: I hear you on that! How would you feel about me making that referral to the nutritionist as a start, and you can then speak to her at your convenience? This is not the same as going to a weight-loss class; she's a specialist in helping cancer survivors and understands the challenges associated with the medications you're taking and the fatigue after treatment.

CASE VIGNETTE

R.B. is a 46-year-old woman who was diagnosed a year ago with cervical cancer. She had a total hysterectomy and chemotherapy. She comes to her transition appointment with the nurse practitioner who runs the survivorship clinic. She is dressed in bright colors with chunky jewelry and makeup to match; her clothing is loose and flowing, and she moves with grace.

When R.B. is asked to get on the scale to be weighed by the nursing assistant, she refuses. She tells the nursing assistant that this appointment has nothing to do with her weight, and she is here only because her oncologist told her that she needed to meet with the nurse practitioner to get her survivorship care plan. She adds that she wants to get this done and be out of the cancer center as quickly as possible.

The nurse practitioner hears the conversation from around the corner and quickly escorts R.B. into her clinic office. It is obvious that the woman is clearly agitated, and any chance of a 60-minute appointment to discuss surveillance and ongoing lifestyle issues is unlikely.

Questions

1. How should the nurse practitioner address R.B.'s refusal to be weighed?
2. Should this be addressed at all? Why or why not?
3. How can the nurse practitioner talk to this woman about maintaining a healthy body weight for optimal outcomes without causing further problems or alienating her?

Conclusion

Talking about weight can be an emotionally laden task for healthcare providers and patients alike. However, not talking about it allows the issue to remain the proverbial elephant in the room. With the current evidence about the association between overweight and obesity and poor outcomes, avoiding weight-related topics could be seen as negligent. This chapter has addressed the issues related to the language used when talking about the topic, as well as the perceived and real barriers for healthcare providers in initiating the conversation. Several models that promote behavior change have also been provided, in addition to examples of how they can be used in talking to patients about their weight and the need for lifestyle changes in those patients who are overweight or obese.

References

Alexander, S.C., Cox, M.E., Turer, C.L.B., Lyna, P., Østbye, T., Tulsky, J.A., … Pollak, K.I. (2011). Do the five A's work when physicians counsel about weight loss? *Family Medicine, 43,* 179–184.

Befort, C.A., Greiner, K.A., Hall, S., Pulvers, K.M., Nollen, N.L., Charbonneau, A., … Ahluwalia, J.S. (2006). Weight-related perceptions among patients and physicians: How well do physicians judge patients' motivation to lose weight? *Journal of General Internal Medicine, 21,* 1086–1090. doi:10.1111/j.1525-1497.2006.00567.x

Bleich, S.N., Bennett, W.L., Gudzune, K.A., & Cooper, L.A. (2012). Impact of physician BMI on obesity care and beliefs. *Obesity, 20,* 999–1005. doi:10.1038/oby.2011.402

Bleich, S.N., Gudzune, K.A., Bennett, W.L., Jarlenski, M.P., & Cooper, L.A. (2013). How does physician BMI impact patient trust and perceived stigma? *Preventive Medicine, 57,* 120–124. doi:10.1016/j.ypmed.2013.05.005

Brown, I., & Thompson., J. (2007). Primary care nurses' attitudes, beliefs, and own body size in relation to obesity management. *Journal of Advanced Nursing, 60,* 535–543. doi:10.1111/j.1365-2648.2007.04450.x

Coa, K.I., Smith, K.C., Klassen, A.C., Caulfield, L.E., Helzlsouer, K., Peairs, K., & Shockney, L. (2015). Capitalizing on the "teachable moment" to promote healthy dietary changes among cancer survivors: The perspectives of health care providers. *Supportive Care in Cancer, 23,* 679–686. doi:10.1007/s00520-014-2412-z

Coa, K.I., Smith, K.C., Klassen, A.C., Thorpe, R.J., Jr., & Caulfield, L.E. (2015). Exploring important influences on the healthfulness of prostate cancer survivors' diets. *Qualitative Health Research, 25,* 857–870. doi:10.1177/1049732315580108

Demark-Wahnefried, W., Aziz, N.M., Rowland, J.H., & Pinto, B.M. (2005). Riding the crest of the teachable moment: Promoting long-term health after the diagnosis of cancer. *Journal of Clinical Oncology, 23,* 5814–5830. doi:10.1200/JCO.2005.01.230

Durant, N.H., Bartman, B., Person, S.D., Collins, F., & Austin, S.B. (2009). Patient provider communication about the health effects of obesity. *Patient Education and Counseling, 75,* 53–57. doi:10.1016/j.pec.2008.09.021

Dutton, G.R., Herman, K.G., Tan, F., Goble, M., Dancer-Brown, M., Van Vessem, N., & Ard, J.D. (2014). Patient and physician characteristics associated with the provision of weight loss counseling in primary care. *Obesity Research and Clinical Practice, 8,* e123–e130. doi:10.1016/j.orcp.2012.12.004

Dutton, G.R., Tan, F., Perri, M.G., Stine, C.C., Dancer-Brown, M., Goble, M., & Van Vessem, N. (2010). What words should we use when discussing excess weight? *Journal of the American Board of Family Medicine, 23,* 606–613. doi:10.3122/jabfm.2010.05.100024

Gudzune, K.A., Beach, M.C., Roter, D.L., & Cooper, L.A. (2013). Physicians build less rapport with obese patients. *Obesity, 21,* 2146–2152. doi:10.1002/oby.20384

Gudzune, K.A., Clark, J.M., Appel, L.J., & Bennett, W.L. (2012). Primary care providers' communication with patients during weight counseling: A focus group study. *Patient Education and Counseling, 89,* 152–157. doi:10.1016/j.pec.2012.06.033

Hash, R.B., Munna, R.K., Vogel, R.L., & Bason, J.J. (2003). Does physician weight affect perception of health advice? *Preventive Medicine, 36,* 41–44. Retrieved from http://www.sciencedirect.com/science/article/pii/S0091743502911242

Humpel, N., Magee, C., & Jones, S.C. (2007). The impact of a cancer diagnosis on the health behaviors of cancer survivors and their family and friends. *Supportive Care in Cancer, 15,* 621–630. doi:10.1007/s00520-006-0207-6

Jay, M., Gillespie, C., Schlair, S., Sherman, S., & Kalet, A. (2010). Physicians' use of the 5As in counseling obese patients: Is the quality of counseling associated with patients' motivation and intention to lose weight? *BMC Health Services Research, 10,* 159. doi:10.1186/1472-6963-10-159

Kable, A., James, C., Snodgrass, S., Plotnikoff, R., Guest, M., Ashby, S., … Collins, C. (2015). Nurse provision of healthy lifestyle advice to people who are overweight or obese. *Nursing and Health Sciences, 17,* 451–459. doi:10.1111/nhs.12214

Kaplan, M. (2010). SPIKES: A framework for breaking bad news to patients with cancer. *Clinical Journal of Oncology Nursing, 14,* 514–516. doi:10.1188/10.CJON.514-516

Lawson, P., & Flocke, S. (2009). Teachable moments for health behavior change: A concept analysis. *Patient Education and Counseling, 76,* 25–30. doi:10.1016/j.pec.2008.11.002

Leske, S., Strodl, E., & Hou, X.-Y. (2012). Patient–practitioner relationships desired by overweight/obese adults. *Patient Education and Counseling, 89,* 309–315. doi:10.1016/j.pec.2012.07.002

Miller, S.K., Alpert, P.T., & Cross, C.L. (2008). Overweight and obesity in nurses, advanced practice nurses, and nurse educators. *Journal of the American Academy of Nurse Practitioners, 20,* 259–265. doi:10.1111/j.1745-7599.2008.00319.x

Pantalon, M.V., Sledge, W.H., Bauer, S.F., Brodsky, B., Giannandrea, S., Kay, J., … Rockland, L.H. (2013). Important medical decisions: Using brief motivational interviewing to enhance patients' autonomous decision-making. *Journal of Psychiatric Practice, 19,* 98–108. doi:10.1097/01.pra.0000428556.48588.22

Pool, A.C., Kraschnewski, J.L., Cover, L.A., Lehman, E.B., Stuckey, H.L., Hwang, K.O., … Sciamanna, C.N. (2014). The impact of physician weight discussion on weight loss in US adults. *Obesity Research and Clinical Practice, 8,* e131–e139. doi:10.1016/j.orcp.2013.03.003

Post, R.E., Mainous, A.G., III, Gregorie, S.H., Knoll, M.E., Diaz, V.A., & Saxena, S.K. (2011). The influence of physician acknowledgment of patients' weight status on patient perceptions of overweight and obesity in the United States. *Archives of Internal Medicine, 171,* 316–321. doi:10.1001/archinternmed.2010.549

Puhl, R.M., Gold, J.A., Luedicke, J., & DePierre, J.A. (2013). The effect of physicians' body weight on patient attitudes: Implications for physician selection, trust and adherence to medical advice. *International Journal of Obesity, 37,* 1415–1421. doi:10.1038/ijo.2013.33

Puhl, R., Peterson, J.L., & Luedicke, J. (2013). Motivating or stigmatizing? Public perceptions of weight-related language used by health providers. *International Journal of Obesity, 37,* 612–619. doi:10.1038/ijo.2012.110

Sinfield, P., Baker, R., Pollard, L., & Tang, M.Y. (2013). Improving the management of obesity in adults: A pilot of a method to identify important barriers to change and tailor interventions to address them. *Quality Primary Care, 21,* 237–246.

Svarovsky, T. (2013). Having difficult conversations: The advanced practitioner's role. *Journal of the Advanced Practitioner in Oncology, 4,* 47–52.

Tailor, A., & Ogden, J. (2009). Avoiding the term 'obesity': An experimental study of the impact of doctors' language on patients' beliefs. *Patient Education and Counseling, 76,* 260–264. doi:10.1016/j.pec.2008.12.016

U.S. Preventive Services Task Force. (2012). Obesity in adults: Screening and management. Retrieved from https://www.uspreventiveservicestaskforce.org/Page/Document/UpdateSummaryFinal/obesity-in-adults-screening-and-management

Chapter 8
Motivational Interviewing

Making lifestyle changes is not easy for anyone—even those who are motivated to change. Most of us have tried at some time in our lives to make some sort of lifestyle change. We may have tried to stop smoking or to reduce our alcohol intake. Even taking a daily multivitamin or calcium can be a challenging change.

It is very hard for our patients to change the way they eat in order to manage their weight. If it were easy, none of our patients would be overweight! Neither would any of us have challenges with our own weight. One technique that might help our patients to make the necessary changes to their eating habits is motivational interviewing (MI). This chapter will explain the basic tenets of this approach and suggest how oncology care providers can use this technique to involve our patients in the decisions that are needed to both accept and change their attitudes and behaviors that are contributing to overweight and obesity.

What Is Motivational Interviewing?

The roots of MI lie in the field of substance abuse counseling. William Miller and Stephen Rollnick published their first book on the topic in 1991. Since then, the technique has moved from addiction counseling to a wide range of other topics, many of them health related. MI was originally proposed as a system of phases. Miller and Rollnick (2013) now describe MI as a technique comprising four processes: engaging, focusing, evoking, and planning. Their work has been widely used and studied and has been modified for use in health promotion and health-related behavior change by multiple authors.

The work of Bruce Berger and William Villaume (2013) is particularly appropriate for understanding how healthcare providers can use MI to encourage change in areas such as adherence to treatment, changes to lifestyle, and management of personal disease. Berger and Villaume suggested that healthcare providers are used to telling patients what to do and providing them with factual information to support our interventions. When patients do not comply with our instructions or appear to not understand what we have told them about their disease or treatment, we blame them for failing to comply with our treatment plan for them. Berger and Villaume suggested that we instead help our patients understand their condition(s) and the options they have for managing their health and then help them to do so.

Patients Are the Experts of Their Own Health

A central tenet of the MI approach is that we are not the only experts in our patients' care. Rather, patients are experts of their life and goals and are responsible for making sense of what we tell them and what they want to do or are capable of doing. This is a challenge for healthcare providers, as many of us have been trained to think of ourselves as the experts as well as the keepers of knowledge. When patients do not follow our instructions or when they question what we tell them to do, we may become defensive, as we interpret this as a challenge to our expertise. It is not easy for many of us to let go of the expert role and allow patients to make decisions. However, holding on to our expert status often results in patients not doing what we advise them to do. This is not a reaction born of ill will but rather the reality of what we tell them to do not fitting in with patients' values, abilities, or interests.

Helping our patients comply with treatment recommendations as well as behavior change is an endeavor that causes healthcare providers significant frustration. Think about how you usually encourage your patients to make changes in their life:

- How often have you thought that the reason a patient did not comply with the treatment plan was because you failed to educate the patient and are therefore responsible in some way? If knowledge was all that it took to change behavior, nobody would smoke. It is common knowledge that smoking causes lung cancer, and yet people, including healthcare providers, smoke!
- Have you ever tried to fix your patients' problems or tried to save them from the consequences of their actions? Because we "know" how to fix health-related problems, we think that it is our role to solve our patients' problems (whether these are because of a lack of motivation to make a change or an apparent inability to follow a treatment plan). Our attempts to save or fix our patients may fail for different reasons. The most important reason is that our patients' problems are not ours to fix. Patients have to solve their own problems, and when we think we can do this for them, we are acting in a paternalistic way. Patients do not like being treated like children, and so they ignore our suggestions (or orders).
- Do you think you can motivate your patients to do what you want them to do or what you think is beneficial for them? When we think it is our responsibility to motivate our patients to make a difficult lifestyle change, we often end up feeling frustrated and angry when patients do not show the expected motivation. This lack of motivation may in reality be a refusal to do what we are telling them to do because they are not ready to make the changes we suggest. We may have wrongly

assumed responsibility for motivation that is internal to them and not something that we can force.

- How often do we characterize patients as "difficult" or "in denial" because they seem resistant to our instructions? It is clear to overweight and obese individuals that they have a problem with their weight. This is not news to them; they have been told this many times by multiple family members, friends, and medical professionals. They look at themselves in the mirror and know this all too well. Many of them will have made multiple efforts to lose weight and perhaps have succeeded for a while and then gained back what they had lost (and more). They are not being difficult and are not in denial when we tell them what they already know. What we label as "denial" is often simply resistance to our efforts because these patients have likely been shamed for their weight before and blamed for it, too. To truly help them, we need to understand the reasons for their resistance. This often affords opportunities to help them in a way that is meaningful and acceptable to them.

Much of what has been described above comes from our acting as if we are central to the patient's health and wellness. Much of what we do in health care is provider centered; we have an agenda or a plan for our interactions with our patients, and these are usually done in an efficient way because we have other patients to see, other teaching sessions to provide, and other meetings and tasks to attend to. When we are provider centered, patients get lost even though we think we are paying attention to them. MI is based on being patient centered, something that many of us think that we practice—but do we really?

Patient-Centeredness: An Underlying Principle of Motivational Interviewing

Berger and Villaume (2013) suggested that the following characteristics exemplify patient-centeredness.

Respecting the patient as a whole person—Our patients are people with values, beliefs, and knowledge about their own bodies that may not be 100% accurate but are the basis of their understanding of their health and illness. Patients are not "cases" or "the breast cancer in Room 3." They have agency (the ability to act on something), and we have a responsibility to respect that and to listen to their thoughts and opinions about their health, even if we disagree with them or think we know more than they do.

Honoring the patient's right to decide—Our patients will decide what information or instructions they agree with. They have the right to decide what they will and will not do. Do not view this as a barrier. If we involve patients in decisions about their health and the care they receive, they will work with us because, ultimately, this is their life to live.

Individualizing care—Patients will decide what they are willing to do to positively affect their health. What works for one person will not necessarily work for another. It is important to remember that telling the patient that other patients have done what you are recommending is not helpful. This is about THIS patient, and being made to feel like one of many other patients is not what the patient wants or needs to motivate change in behavior.

Personalizing care—This means finding out what has meaning for patients. We do this by asking what would encourage patients to make a change in what they do or to adhere to the treatment plan. By asking these types of questions, we can learn what the facilitators and barriers to change are for each individual patient.

Shared decision making—Because patients are ultimately responsible for their own health, dictating what they must do is counterproductive. We can provide patients with information about their health and resources to help them manage their illness, but this should be offered as one of a number of options and not as an order.

A sense of safety and care—When care is patient centered, the individual will feel cared for, respected, valued, and safe. In this context, patients are more likely to listen to what we have to say, consider the options available to them, and work with us to optimize their health and wellness.

Motivational Interviewing in Health Care

Even though many healthcare providers truly believe that we are patient centered and uphold the characteristics mentioned in the previous section, the reality is that we think we do more than we actually do. Although we may see each patient as a whole person, honor the patient's right to decide what should happen, think that we individualize and personalize care and promote shared decision making, and strive to care for our patients safely, in reality, we care for our patients in a busy and time-pressured context. Some of us have just 15 minutes for each interaction with our patients. Others have even less time and rush from one patient to another, barely managing to assess their physical status and with no time at all to get to know them as individuals with a set of values and beliefs. Some of us rely on printed materials or a list of online resources to educate our patients because we do not have time for face-to-face discussions, and this may be better than nothing at all. Some of us operate on autopilot; we have a set of messages for our patients and everyone gets the same message with no individualization of information and no assessment of what they already know or interest in what they are prepared or able to do to improve their health. Then we wonder why our patients do not listen or adhere to our instructions!

Many of us have learned to talk to our patients in ways that are not conducive to their understanding. We may use medical terms (or even Latin names for diseases or body parts) or talk in "nurse speak," an abbreviated manner of speaking that sounds much like the brief notes we make in patient records. We may use jargon and talk very fast, not bothering to check if our patients understand what we are saying. Although our patients may be sitting quietly and nodding, this does NOT mean that they understand. They may not want to interrupt the flow of the lecture we are giving, may not want to appear stupid, or may be afraid to ask questions or to request that we repeat or clarify what we have told them. These patients then leave the clinic or office not fully understanding what we have instructed them to do, therefore failing to adhere to our instructions. So the next time we see them, we try harder to get our message across and that may mean talking louder or more forcefully, ultimately making these patients feel like failures while it is WE who have failed to communicate in a way that our patients understand.

Communication comprises two dimensions: content (what we say) and relational (how we talk and how it is received). The content of our communication with patients is influenced by the relational dimension; nonverbal messages such as tone, facial expression, and gestures underlie the relational aspects of communication and can "speak" loudly. A power differential exists between patients and their healthcare providers. Healthcare providers traditionally possess knowledge, expertise, and authority over patients. When our patients do not do what they have been told to do, we interpret this as resistance.

Relational Resistance

There may be patient resistance to aspects of the relational dimension of communication. This relates to who holds power and autonomy in the patient–provider relationship. If healthcare providers act as if they know what is best and assume that they know more than their patients, relational resistance may occur. Patients will feel as if they have lost face and will resist listening and reacting in a constructive manner. We all want to feel as though we can make independent decisions about our own life and health. When someone tells us what to do or implies that we are stupid because we did not do what we were told, we "lose face," or feel humiliated or disrespected. We feel embarrassed and diminished and act with resistance to the message in order to assert ourselves and regain a sense of power. This is a subconscious process and not something patients intentionally do.

Issue Resistance

Patients who do not appear to be adhering to our recommendations may not hold the same understanding of the issue and thus resist based on their own understanding and reasoning. Even though their reasoning may not be factually correct, it makes sense to them; they see little reason to change their behavior. For example, patients who do not understand the link between overweight and obesity and cancer recurrence may resist our recommendation to lose weight. In their reasoning, losing weight is suggestive of being sick from treatment or the cancer recurring, and if they do not look "sick," then they must be OK. This is an example of practical reasoning, which is part of issue resistance. If we tell patients that this reasoning is not valid, then they may lose face, causing additional relational resistance.

Sense Making

To change some aspect of their behavior, patients must make sense of why it is important. Being diagnosed with a life-threatening illness like cancer is a pivotal experience for most people. It usually results in people wanting to make changes in their life, in part as a way of making sense of why they got cancer and also in an attempt to prevent cancer recurrence. MI capitalizes on these aspects of the patient's experience.

A lifestyle change after cancer may make sense to some patients, and this may be reinforced by family and friends who desperately want their loved one to survive and recover. The patient and family will attempt to align their understanding and knowledge about the cancer with what the patient values and has confidence that he or she can do to mitigate the consequences of the disease and treatments. This is termed *practical reasoning*; the healthcare provider can use this reasoning to help patients want to make the necessary health behavior changes without imposing their own reasoning onto their patients. To impose our own reasoning on patients risks the development of resistance.

Now that you have read about the underpinnings of MI—patients as the experts of their own life and health, patient-centeredness, resistance to our message, and sense making—how do we proceed?

Steps in Motivational Interviewing

This chapter in no way does justice to the practice of MI. MI is an approach that requires understanding beyond the few pages in this chapter. Practice in a workshop setting and real-world experience with patients are essential. It is not easy for many healthcare providers to adapt to and adopt the techniques described in MI. Our education, training, and practice places us in opposition to much of what MI is about. Most of us have been led to believe that we are the experts and that we are in charge of our patients along their disease and treatment trajectory. We are used to giving direct instructions to patients and expect them to follow these instructions. We often think that patient recommendations are based on evidence and are not influenced by our own preferences, assumptions, and biases.

MI is based on the idea that patients are the experts of their own life and health. Healthcare providers can guide patients to a better understanding of their health or disease, but it is the patients' decision on what to follow. We bring our own feelings, attitudes, and values to the interaction with our patients, and this may act as a barrier when they oppose the feelings, attitudes, and beliefs of our patients.

The six steps of MI are as follows: develop rapport, reframe the issue, ask permission to provide more information, provide new information, ask patients what they think of the new information, and summarize and discuss next steps.

Develop Rapport

Rapport is developed with patients when we listen to them and then reflect our understanding of what they think, understand, and feel about what they have been told. This needs to be done in a respectful manner and with no judgment. When patients respond to the question about what they have understood from the information provided to them, healthcare providers can actively listen and assess whether their patients are motivated to make changes—and if not, why. Is any lack of motivation due to their patients' perception that the change is not important? Do they lack the confidence that they can make the change? Or, is the lack of motivation attributable to a combination of these two reasons?

Developing rapport involves the development of trust, and we do this by paying attention to what our patients are saying, by listening to them in a nonjudgmental way, and by not scolding them when they do not do what we tell them to do. When we accurately reflect on what our patients have shared with us about their understanding and feelings, and when we actively involve them in decision making and do not impose our views and goals on them, rapport is established.

Listening and empathetic response are key elements in building trust and rapport with our patients. Listening is an active process (different from hearing, which is passive) and involves paying attention and avoiding distraction. Many distractions exist in healthcare environments; pagers, cell phones, note taking by hand or on a tablet or computer, and general multitasking tells our patients that we are not really paying attention. A barrier to active listening is interrupting patients (often to ask for additional information or to correct something they have said). Our own mental processes, such as evaluating what our patients have said, judging them, trying to mentally fix their problems, or making assumptions about what and how they are feeling, also are barriers to active listening. When we are distracted, we give the message that our patients are not important or of value; this causes relational resistance. When we correct our patients, we cause content resistance.

When we listen to patients, we are able to respond empathetically. This helps patients to feel less alone or isolated. When we respond empathetically to patients, we build a therapeutic alliance. In this relationship, patients learn from their healthcare provider. In turn, healthcare providers learn about their patients, including their experience of their illness and their willingness to make changes in their lifestyle.

An empathetic response is not the same as stating that you understand what your patient is going through or feeling. An empathetic response reflects that you validate how your patient is feeling, the reason why your patient is feeling that way, and what he or she is experiencing. Empathetic responses do not involve a generalized statement about how others feel in a similar situation; this has no meaning for the patient and may make them feel worse when they think they are being compared to others. An empathetic response does not include talking about oneself, even if you have experienced something similar to your patient.

Reframe the Issue

Healthcare providers seek to provide clarification to their patients about any issues or misunderstandings, thus allowing their patients to see things differently or to make sense of things in a different way. One way that healthcare providers can reframe the issue for a patient is to ask the patient what he or she knows or thinks about the issue and then tailor a response that is empathetic and takes into account the patient's knowledge and attitude. Many patients know they need to lose weight and have tried, often repeatedly. The issue here is not that the patient has failed at losing weight; rather, it is that the patient has not been able to maintain the weight loss. Reframing the issue from failing to lose weight to maintaining the weight loss puts it in a new perspective and allows the patient to feel encouraged about any previous success (losing weight) and to focus on ways to maintain future weight-loss efforts. Another way of reframing an issue is to ask patients what life would be like if they were successful at making these necessary lifestyle changes. This is called "looking over the fence" and allows patients to imagine what life would be like if they were successful in changing their behavior. In responding to the scenario, patients create their own benefits; these are usually personally meaningful and may increase their motivation and commitment to making the change.

Ask Permission to Provide More Information

Healthcare providers should ask permission to provide patients with new information. We cannot assume that our patients want more information or are ready to hear new information.

Once you have an understanding of what your patients know about the role of overweight and obesity in cancer and how they have made sense of this in the context of their life, it may be appropriate to provide patients with new information to correct myths or misunderstandings. Merely giving new information, often while interrupting patients, can make them defensive and resistant to hearing the information we are in a hurry to provide. "Lecturing" patients causes them to feel stupid or like a child and ultimately to lose face.

Asking respectfully if we can provide "new" information (rather than "correct" information) is more likely to encourage patients to listen actively. An example of how to ask permission is to use a phrase such as, "Can I tell you what worries me about your belief that additional weight is not harmful?" This identifies that you want to talk about something specific and that you are also being respectful in asking if the patient wants to hear your concern. If the patient says that they do not want to talk about this, unless the situation is immediately harmful to the patient, you should respect that. In your response, provide the information in a nondirective way. For example, you could respond with, "It is your decision whether you want to learn more about the role that being overweight plays in the recurrence of cancer. I know that you are worried about this and are trying to do everything you can to prevent this from happening. Any amount of weight that you lose during survivorship is helpful in preventing the cancer from coming back, and I want to help to keep you as healthy as possible."

Provide New Information

New information must address aspects of patients' sense making and must provide patients with an opportunity to reconsider how they are making sense of the situation.

Remember that it is through sense making that patients are motivated to change their behavior (not just by us providing them with additional information).

Phrases such as, "You need to understand that . . ." or "Don't you know that . . ." are prescriptive and judgmental; they make patients feel stupid and increase resistance. Simple statements of fact, in neutral and plain language, are more likely to be received by patients. An example of a simple statement for a patient who fears that weight loss is suggestive of being sick is, "Being overweight increases your risk of the breast cancer coming back." This feels more neutral than a prescriptive statement that includes medical jargon (recurrence), such as, "You don't want your cancer to recur, do you? If you don't lose weight, you are increasing your risk of recurrence."

Ask Patients What They Think of the New Information

Seeking an answer to the question "What do you think about that?" allows us to assess what the next steps might be based on what our patients understand or feel about what they have been told. It also will help us learn what additional information our patients may need. By asking our patients for their thoughts on this new information, we also learn if the information we have provided has influenced our patients and helped them understand what they need to do to make changes in their lifestyle and behaviors.

Instances may occur where patients still are not ready to make the changes you think are necessary. They may need more time to think about what they have been told and may not fully "buy in" to what they need to do—or, they simply may not be ready to make a change. By voicing acceptance of this, you are letting your patients know that you are hopeful that they will make the change in their behavior and that you are willing to talk to them at another time. An example of a response to patients who say that they do not agree with your recommendations might be, "I can hear that you are still not sure of the importance of your present weight to your cancer recovery. What else do you need to know about how to manage this?"

This can be frustrating for all; your patients feel pressured to do something that they may not be fully ready to do, and you feel that you have done everything to inform your patients while respecting their autonomy. Showing frustration is not helpful. It is always important to remember that despite our best attempts, our patients have the right to decide how to live their lives—even if we think we know better!

Summarize and Discuss Next Steps

The final step is to summarize what you understand about your patients' thinking now that information has been provided. It is not an opportunity to summarize what you have told your patients but rather a reflection on what your patients have told you about their understanding and their motivation. Then, ask your patients what they want to do next.

For many patients, this is when they feel overwhelmed and unsure of exactly what they need to do. It can be helpful to provide them with options and reassurance that they are not alone and that you will help them as they institute the changes into their daily life. An example of how to suggest this would be, "There are two or three ways to start on a weight-loss plan. You can increase the amount of exercise you get every day. You can change how and when you eat. Or, you can do both. What you decide to do is up to you, and I will help you in any way I can."

Challenges

Although the information provided in this chapter may seem simple, it is not. Most healthcare providers have been trained to be directive, to ask questions in a predictable (to us) manner, and to focus on what we need to know to make a diagnosis or elicit information about our patients and their diseases. MI requires a change of mindset as well as a different way of communicating.

Not all patients want to change, and our attempts to inform and encourage them may result in anger. This can cause us to get angry and frustrated in response or to engage in blaming and shaming. Once that type of thinking happens, any chance of a therapeutic relationship being created or maintained between the patient and healthcare provider is lost. Anger in patients often is a result of feeling powerless. Cancer is a scary disease for many, and past experiences of cancer in family members or friends will color their perception, despite what we tell them about survival statistics. Powerlessness also can result from patients' perception that their care is substandard—that the diagnostic process has been delayed or that they have had to wait past their appointment times to see healthcare providers. Patients may be tired after an extended series of waits for procedures and tests. They then have to sit and talk about their weight, a topic that makes them uncomfortable.

It also can be challenging for overweight or obese healthcare providers to talk about the need for their patients to manage their weight. It is important to note that patients may think (and say outright) that it is hypocritical for their healthcare provider to suggest that they need to manage their weight when it is obvious that the healthcare provider cannot. An appropriate response for healthcare providers is to acknowledge their own struggles but to be careful about sharing too much personal information so that the focus does not move to them instead of remaining on their patient.

The Evidence on Motivational Interviewing and Weight Loss

The role of MI in weight-loss counseling has been explored in a few studies, but none involved a cancer population. Armstrong et al. (2011) conducted a systematic review and meta-analysis and concluded that MI resulted in greater weight loss compared to controls in overweight and obese individuals. A more recent systematic review and meta-analysis found that as little as one MI session may be effective for creating behavior change in the clinical setting (VanBuskirk & Wetherell, 2014). Barnes and

Ivezaj (2015) reviewed 19 studies and concluded that most studies do not report on MI fidelity. However, of the studies they reviewed, 13 reported weight loss of at least 5% of initial body weight and 9 reported significant weight loss compared to controls. DiLillo and West (2011) noted that some studies showed inconsistent weight loss in participants and questioned whether the training of the providers of the MI intervention was sufficient. In a study of physician use of MI techniques when counseling overweight or obese patients, those patients who perceived their physician to be empathetic were more satisfied with their care and more confident that they could lose weight (Pollak et al., 2011).

When physicians use MI techniques (empathy, encouragement of a physician–patient partnership, avoidance of directive language, reflection and open-ended questions), patients reported greater confidence in their ability to improve their nutritional status and ate more fiber and less fat (Cox et al., 2011). Patients also lost weight when they were counseled by physicians using MI techniques compared to those whose physicians did not use language that was empathetic and reflective (Pollak et al., 2010). In one study, female physicians were more likely to use MI techniques with their patients than their male counterparts (54% vs. 41%) (Pollak et al., 2011). Only one study reflecting nursing practice was found (Östlund, Kristofferzon, Häggström, & Wadensten, 2015), and this showed that none of the primary nurses achieved beginning proficiency in the use of MI techniques when counseling patients on lifestyle changes, despite using these techniques on patients aged 2–11 years.

CASE VIGNETTE

L.K. is a 63-year-old woman and has recently completed chemotherapy for left-sided breast cancer that is estrogen receptor, progesterone receptor, and HER2 positive. She had a unilateral mastectomy prior to starting chemotherapy.

At L.K.'s treatment completion appointment, the nurse practitioner (NP) presents L.K. with a survivorship care plan. They discuss what steps she should take to keep healthy in the years to come. L.K. becomes tearful when the NP mentions that it is important to maintain a healthy weight. The NP stops talking about the survivorship care plan and, using the six steps of MI, begins a discussion with L.K. about weight management after breast cancer treatment.

Develop Rapport

NP: You're upset about something I said concerning maintaining a healthy weight. Are you willing to share with me what is making you so upset?

L.K.: I've just been through so much in the past 18 months with the surgery and the chemotherapy, and now I have to take tamoxifen. Everything I read about it says that I am going to gain even more weight. I can't handle that!

NP: You think that you will gain weight while taking tamoxifen. That must be frustrating for you on top of everything that you've gone through during treatment.

L.K.: Yes, it is frustrating. It's the story of my life. I've always been heavy, even as a teenager. And I've tried repeatedly to lose the weight. I was the thinnest I have ever been at my wedding. Then, I put on weight with my first pregnancy, and before I knew it, I was pregnant again. Believe me, getting off the "baby weight" was not easy with two kids under two years of age! I never really lost all of that weight, and now it's going to be impossible! My husband had a heart attack five years ago, and I have to watch him in case it happens again. I also help my daughter with her two children, and that's not easy. How am I supposed to do all that AND lose all this weight?

Reframe the Issue

NP: It sounds like you have been busy caring for everyone else and have not had the time to take care of yourself. How do you think your life might be different if you lost some weight?

L.K.: Well, I don't know. How much would I have to lose? I'm not sure how much I weigh or even how much I've put on over the years. I never weigh myself, and I ask the nurses not to tell me what the scale says when they weigh me at my appointments. I guess I'm in denial. I can't even tell if my clothes are tight because I wear loose dresses so that no one can see that my boobs are lopsided.

Ask Permission to Provide New Information

NP: Can we talk about what is a healthy weight for you? Perhaps after that, we can see if you are interested in hearing about how you can plan to eat healthy foods and manage any extra weight without putting any more stress on you.

L.K.: Well, OK, I guess. It's just that I don't have much time to shop and cook and everything. It's as if I have two full-time jobs: my husband and my grandkids.

Provide New Information

NP: When making any kind of change to lifestyle, it's important to bear in mind what is possible for you to do. Your life is really busy. Eating a healthy diet would be good for your husband, too, after his heart attack. It's also good for your grandchildren. I am going to suggest some small changes that you can make that won't require a lot of extra work and that will help all of you to eat more healthily. To start with, let's talk about what you prepare and eat every day.

L.K.: We don't really eat breakfast. The kids sometimes ask for cereal when they get back from nursery and kindergarten around noon, and I usually have some with them. Just before my daughter comes to pick them up at about 5 o'clock, we have some juice and cookies. Then my husband and I usually get something from the drive-thru, or I just make some pasta with sauce. I'm really tired by then—we often don't sit down to eat until 7:30 or 8 pm—and dinner has to be quick, or else I'm falling asleep in my plate!

NP: You have a lot going on in your day. You must be starving by noon, and although cereal is quick and easy, and the grandkids like it, it doesn't have much protein or fiber. One area where you can make a real change is by eating breakfast regularly; some eggs or oatmeal are good choices. Having some fruit and cheese when your grandchildren are there will keep them fueled for an afternoon of play, and that's a good lunch for you and your husband.

Ask the Patient What She Thinks of the New Information

NP: What do you think about the suggestions I've made about eating breakfast and also about including more protein and fruit for your lunch with your grandchildren?

L.K.: I think I could do that. It will be weird to have to cook breakfast, and I don't know if eggs are healthy for my husband. I guess it wouldn't hurt the kids to have something other than cereal when they are at our house. They eat those "cheese string things" at their house, and I could get some of those.

Summarize and Discuss Next Steps

NP: It's great that you're willing to make these changes, even though making breakfast is going to be a change for you. Including more protein and fruit will be good for your grandchildren, too. I understand your concern for your husband's health; we have to take that into consideration. There are other things that you could do, too. Do you want to talk about those now or leave them for another day? I also can refer you to our nutritionist, who will have a lot of tips and helpful hints to keep you on track.

Example of a Negative Conversation With the Same Patient

NP: I need to talk to you about your weight. You really need to lose weight to prevent a recurrence of your cancer. Do you have any idea how much weight you've gained since you started treatment?

L.K.: I don't know what I weigh, and I don't want to know. That just upsets me, and I don't need to be upset right now. This has been really hard for me. My husband had a heart attack five years ago, and I look after my two grandchildren, too.

NP: This has nothing to do with your husband, but I bet he could stand to lose some weight, too. All you have to do is eat less and exercise more and you'll lose weight. It's really quite simple.

L.K.: I've tried and tried to lose weight and nothing helps.

NP: Well, maybe you don't realize that you are taking a big risk with your life. If your cancer recurs, it may be too late to do anything. Metastatic cancer is not curable, you know.

[L.K. starts to cry]

NP: I'm sorry to upset you, but you need to know the truth. This is serious.

L.K.: Don't you think I know this is serious? Don't you think I've tried? I need to help my family, but this is so hard.

In this example of poor communication, the NP is not actively listening to what L.K. is saying. She shows no empathy and does not consider how the patient makes sense of what she is being told or why she needs to eat more healthily. The NP uses scare tactics, medical language, and a threatening tone that overwhelms and frightens the patient. L.K. is progressively getting more upset and is not able to listen to what she is being told, even though there is little in the way of constructive information provided to her.

Conclusion

MI is designed to help patients verbalize the personal reasons behind why they want to lose weight as well as to talk about why they may not be able to do so. MI encourages discussion about ambivalence toward making the lifestyle changes necessary to lose or maintain weight, along with exploration of the obstacles they may encounter when they attempt to make these changes.

Although it may appear easy to use MI techniques in everyday practice, caution should be used. This technique requires training, practice, and skill to be effective. Resources for additional information about MI are provided at the end of this chapter. Although most of the evidence suggests that MI is a valid and useful approach, it should not be seen as a panacea that will work for all patients. It is, however, well worth including in your practice in talking to patients about weight control.

Resources

- Motivational Interviewing Network of Trainers (MINT) is an international organization that provides training and resources for MI providers: www.motivationalinterviewing.org
- YouTube offers various instructional videos on MI techniques that healthcare providers can apply to their training and practice: www.youtube.com/results?=motivational+interviewing

References

Armstrong, M.J., Mottershead, T.A., Ronksley, P.E., Sigal, R.J., Campbell, T.S., & Hemmelgarn, B.R. (2011). Motivational interviewing to improve weight loss in overweight and/or obese patients: A systematic review and meta-analysis of randomized controlled trials. *Obesity Review, 12,* 709–723. doi:10.1111/j.1467-789X.2011.00892.x

Barnes, R.D., & Ivezaj, V. (2015). A systematic review of motivational interviewing for weight loss among adults in primary care. *Obesity Review, 16,* 304–318. doi:10.1111/obr.12264

Berger, B.A., & Villaume, W.A. (2013). *Motivational interviewing for health care professionals: A sensible approach.* Washington, DC: American Pharmacists Association.

Cox, M.E., Yancy, W.S., Jr., Coffman, C.J., Østbye, T., Tulsky, J.A., Alexander, S.C., … Pollak, K.I. (2011). Effects of counseling techniques on patients' weight-related attitudes and behaviors in a primary care clinic. *Patient Education and Counseling, 85,* 363–368. doi:10.1016/j.pec.2011.01.024

DiLillo, V., & West, D.S. (2011). Motivational interviewing for weight loss. *Psychiatric Clinics of North America, 34,* 861–869. doi:10.1016/j.psc.2011.08.003

Miller, W.E., & Rollnick, S. (2013). *Motivational interviewing: Helping people change* (3rd ed.). New York, NY: Guilford Press.

Östlund, A.-S., Kristofferzon, M.-L., Häggström, E., & Wadensten, B. (2015). Primary care nurses' performance in motivational interviewing: A quantitative descriptive study. *BMC Family Practice, 16,* 1–12. doi:10.1186/s12875-015-0304-z

Pollak, K.I., Alexander, S.C., Coffman, C.J., Tulsky, J.A., Lyna, P., Dolor, R.J., … Østbye, T. (2010). Physician communication techniques and weight loss in adults: Project CHAT. *American Journal of Preventive Medicine, 39,* 321–328. doi:10.1016/j.amepre.2010.06.005

Pollak, K.I., Coffman, C.J., Alexander, S.C., Manusov, J.R., Østbye, T., Tulsky, J.A., … Dolor, R.J. (2011). Predictors of weight loss communication in primary care encounters. *Patient Education and Counseling, 85,* e175–e182. doi:10.1016/j.pec.2011.03.001

VanBuskirk, K.A., & Wetherell, J.L. (2014). Motivational interviewing with primary care populations: A systematic review and meta-analysis. *Journal of Behavioral Medicine, 37,* 768–780. doi:10.1007/s10865-013-9527-4

Chapter 9
Mindfulness and Overweight and Obesity

Given the adverse consequences of overweight and obesity on recurrence and poor outcomes in cancer, finding ways to help survivors prevent weight gain or control their weight is important. One way of doing this may be using mindfulness-based interventions. This chapter will provide a brief overview of mindfulness and how it is used in reducing physical and psychological effects of illness, including cancer. The evidence on mindfulness-based interventions targeting weight control will be described, and resources for providers and patients will be listed at the end of the chapter. Related topics, including intuitive and mindful eating, will be briefly discussed.

Mindfulness

Mindfulness as a movement or philosophy began as a form of Buddhist meditation nearly 4,000 years ago. Jon Kabat-Zinn is a pioneer in the field of mindfulness in health care. His research and writing have led to the development of therapies such as mindfulness-based stress reduction (MBSR) and mindfulness-based cognitive therapy (MBCT) (Brotto & Goldmeier, 2015). MBSR is more commonly used with physical manifestations of illness, and MBCT with cognitive aspects (Gotink et al., 2015).

Kabat-Zinn describes *mindfulness* as the awareness that comes from paying attention to something on purpose and in the present moment with an attitude of nonjudgment (Paulson, Davidson, Jha, & Kabat-Zinn, 2013). This does not mean that people have to forgo judgment to be mindful but rather to not judge themselves about how judgmental they are! In practice, this means ignoring the thoughts, opinions, and negative judgments we think about constantly. This is particularly relevant when it comes to food, with so many of us judging food as either "good" or "bad." Good foods are healthy like fruits and vegetables; bad foods are the ones we crave such as chocolate, candies, and pastries.

Mindfulness is not a religion or belief system. It is a means of maintaining awareness from moment to moment without distraction and with the intent of creating emotional balance and a sense of well-being (Ludwig & Kabat-Zinn, 2008). The practice of mindfulness has been used by Kabat-Zinn and others in the treatment of different conditions, including stress, pain, and coping (Ludwig & Kabat-Zinn, 2008). Kabat-Zinn's stress reduction program comprises eight sessions (one session per week). Each session is 150 minutes long. The sessions include lectures, formal meditation practice, yoga, and a six-hour silent meditation retreat. Meditation at home is an essential part of the program, as is the practice of mindfulness during usual daily activities. Many of the interventions used in clinical trials as described in this chapter are modifications of this program and include one or more components (not the full spectrum as designed for the formal program).

Mindfulness in Cancer

Mindfulness-based interventions have been used extensively in cancer populations—primarily in women with breast cancer and secondly in men with prostate cancer. In an overview of meta-analyses and systematic reviews of the effectiveness of mindfulness-based interventions in a total of 1,668 cancer survivors, significant improvements were seen in anxiety, stress, depression, and overall quality of life (Gotink et al., 2015). A dose–response relationship was evident. Improvement in mood was associated with the amount of time spent meditating. Stress reduction was associated with the number of sessions attended.

Rouleau, Garland, and Carlson (2015) conducted a review of mindfulness-based interventions for individuals with cancer and concluded that methodologic concerns were present with many of the studies. Of note is that in evaluating the influence of mindfulness on psychological distress, self-report measures have been used rather than validated measures or formal diagnostic procedures. Inclusion criteria for the studies have not screened for those with preintervention distress. Mindfulness-based interventions for sleep also have methodologic issues similar to the interventions previously described. With these caveats in mind, sleep quality, sleep latency, wake after sleep onset, and insomnia have all been shown to improve following mindfulness-based interventions. The review concluded that mindfulness-based interventions improve cancer-related fatigue. Evidence also exists, most often from small, single-arm studies, that mindfulness-based interventions improve various aspects of psychological health, including comfort, happiness, post-traumatic growth, and positive affect.

An earlier review suggested that mindfulness-based interventions can improve mood and quality of life and reduce distress in people with cancer; however, this meta-analysis also suggested that larger studies with adequate control and longer follow-up are needed to show efficacy of these interventions (Musial, Büssing, Heusser, Choi, & Ostermann, 2011). This is echoed in another systematic review and meta-analysis in women with breast cancer, which suggested that MBSR is effective for improving psychological health for these women (Cramer, Lauche, Paul, & Dobos, 2012); however, more robust studies are needed.

A meta-analysis on the benefits of MBSR in women with breast cancer concluded that quality of life and psychological functioning improve when women participate in MBSR interventions (Huang, He, Wang, & Zhou, 2016). MBSR has been shown to increase telomere activity in women with breast cancer but not telomere length (Lengacher et al., 2014). Both telomere length and activity are markers of cellular aging and oxidative stress and may be affected by psychological distress. In this study, telomere activity increased by 17%, compared to 3% in the control group. Although the differences were not significantly correlated with changes in mindfulness, other psychological measures, or the amount of meditation practice, the findings were consistent with previous studies demonstrating increased telomere activity following stress-reducing interventions. Telomere length is seen to need at least one year to show signs of change; therefore, this 12-week study period may not have been long enough to show a change in this marker.

Mindfulness and Overweight and Obesity

Mindfulness-based interventions targeting obesity have become increasingly popular over the past few years in noncancer populations. Many overweight and obese individuals are known to eat "mindlessly." They eat fast, often in front of the television or computer or while doing other activities, and are not mindful, or aware, of what or how much they are eating (Rubin, 2014). This can cause chronic overeating, weight gain, and poor blood glucose control, leading to the development of diabetes and other chronic and serious health conditions. Some people are "emotional eaters" and use food to temporarily reduce their stress or distress; given that cancer itself is a significant source of stress, overeating may be a coping mechanism for individuals with cancer and lead to overweight and obesity.

Stress is theorized to activate the hypothalamic–pituitary–adrenal axis, resulting in high levels of cortisol production. This hormone binds to fat cells and activates lipoprotein lipase, which converts triglycerides into free fatty acids in adipocytes. In combination with insulin, amino acids and fatty acids are sent to the abdomen so that the liver can use them to provide energy for the brain.

In a randomized controlled trial, obese individuals who participated in a four-month mindfulness-based program targeting stress eating showed significant reductions in cortisol awakening response and maintained their weight (Daubenmier et al., 2011). The intervention created mindfulness, and participants showed more awareness of body sensations of hunger and satiety and reduced their consumption of foods in response to emotions.

An intensive 10-week program comprising 90-minute sessions targeting food cravings was studied by other researchers. This intervention was based on acceptance of the sensations of food cravings. When participants experienced food cravings, they were instructed to let these feelings pass and not act on them immediately. The intervention showed success in lowering cravings, decreasing obsession with food, and lowering the extent to which participants experienced loss of control when presented with food cues (Alberts, Mulkens, Smeets, & Thewissen, 2010).

Food cues are an important aspect of what, when, and how much we eat. In a novel experiment using a "bottomless bowl," a soup bowl that automatically refilled itself, participants who ate from these bowls consumed 14.7 oz of soup versus 8.5 oz for those who had normal bowls (Wansink, Painter, & North, 2005). This equaled 73% more food eaten and an additional 113 calories. The researchers concluded that we use visual cues to estimate how much we have eaten rather than using physical cues of fullness or feeling satiated. This is associated with the phenomenon of "cleaning our plates" rather than ceasing consumption when we feel satiated. This is of particular significance in today's world, where restaurant and fast food portions are much larger than they used to be, and cleaning one's plate means consuming large amounts of excessive food and calories.

A six-week intervention called Mindful Eating and Living (MEAL) was tested in another study, where participants attended weekly sessions comprising training in mindfulness meditation as well as group discussion with daily homework (Dalen et al., 2010). When compared to baseline, participants in the MEAL program showed statistically significant increases in mindfulness and cognitive restraint with eating and also statistically significant weight loss, less disinhibited eating (eating when full), less binge eating, and decreased depression. The authors suggested that mindfulness promotes attention to physical cues of fullness and internal dialogues, and, as a result, eating patterns can be changed.

In another study, a single one-hour training session in mindfulness resulted in 86% of participants eating healthy food. More than 60% of participants noted that they paid more attention to various aspects of the meal they ate after the training, including the appearance, taste, and texture of the food, the size of the bites they took, and their feelings of calmness (Jacobs, Cardaciotto, Block-Lerner, & McMahon, 2013). This study suggests that there might be utility in a short mindfulness training for immediate effects; however, how long and effectively this could be maintained is an important question.

A pilot study of 11 weekly classes on nutrition that used mindfulness training was conducted with men with prostate cancer (Carmody et al., 2012). The classes promoted a dietary change that included more vegetables than animal proteins in the participants' diets. Although this is thought to be protective for prostate cancer risk, the effects of this dietary change on men with prostate cancer are more likely related to their risk of cardiovascular disease. The men's partners were included in the classes, as it was recognized that they play a significant role in buying and preparing food. Three months after the class, the intervention group maintained the dietary change of more vegetables than animal proteins. This was significantly associated with mindfulness training.

Self-compassion is an element of mindfulness; it is a way of relating to oneself with kindness and nonjudgment (Mantzios & Wilson, 2013). In a study of 243 healthy students, mindfulness and self-compassion predicted weight loss. Self-compassion alone helped with maintenance of weight, and mindfulness alone was associated with weight loss. A combination of the two resulted in increased weight loss. This may have relevance to individuals who are constantly attempting to lose weight and who tend to judge themselves harshly when they "slip up" and either gain weight or go off their diets. Being less self-critical may be more helpful than constantly judging oneself and trying over and over to lose weight.

A review of mindfulness-based interventions on obesity and related eating behaviors concluded that of the 21 studies reviewed, 86% showed improvements in eating behaviors such as binge eating, emotional eating, and eating in response to external cues such as the appearance and smell of food rather than on hunger cues (O'Reilly, Cook, Spruijt-Metz, & Black, 2014). The authors pointed out that many studies on mindfulness interventions and obesity and eating behaviors are conducted within a population of Caucasian students. Cultural and ethnic diversity is needed to make the conclusions relevant and more applicable to the real world.

Mindful Eating

The amount we eat is under our control, and *mindful eating*, eating with awareness of physical and emotional sensations, has been shown to modify how much we eat, our ability to self-regulate our eating to increase weight loss, and the psychological distress related to obesity. Beshara, Hutchinson, and Wilson (2013) studied the effects of self-reported everyday mindfulness and serving sizes of energy-dense foods such as pastries, jams and sweet spreads, savory pastries, fast foods, chocolate, ice cream, cookies, and candy. Mindful eaters reported smaller portions of these energy-dense foods and less emotional eating. They also ate less when full and were aware of satiety and hunger sensations, resulting in eating smaller portions. The authors suggested that including training in mindful eating may be a useful addition to weight-loss strategies for the role that mindful eating plays in reducing serving sizes.

An eight-week mindful eating intervention was evaluated in a small group of obese women (Kidd, Graor, & Murrock, 2013). The only measurable increase was seen in self-efficacy for weight loss; however, qualitative data from this study showed some interesting benefits of the intervention and subsequent practice of mindful eating. Initially, the women in the study found that being more mindful of what they were eating was burdensome. However, over time they began to feel in control of what and how they ate, and this resulted in emotional gains such as feeling happier and less depressed. The women became more aware of the changes they were making in food choices and also of self-sabotaging thoughts and behaviors. They also found being in a group to be helpful and supportive and felt it their responsibility to members of the group to attain the goals they had set for themselves.

Mindful attention has been shown to mitigate the effects of hunger on how attractive unhealthy food appears and the choices made by individuals. It also has been shown to reduce food cravings (Papies, Pronk, Keesman, & Barsalou, 2015). It is suggested that mindful attention allows individuals to recognize that thoughts are merely fleeting events and do not need to be acted on. It also is suggested that mindful attention reduces how attractive food appears to be. Individuals are able to control their behavior, and the anticipation of a "reward" (unhealthy food) is mitigated by self-control.

What Does It Mean to Be a Mindful Eater?

In essence, mindful eating is not about intensive training sessions or lengthy instruction manuals but rather an approach to eating that is slow and attentive to taste, hunger, and satiety (Mathieu, 2009). Mindful eating does not place any restrictions on type of food, amount of food, timing of consumption, or location of meals. Mindful eating involves eating more slowly and away from distractions such as the TV or in the car, using physical cues such as hunger and fullness to start and stop eating, not judging food likes and dislikes, using all senses while eating, appreciating food that is nourishing and pleasant to eat, and being aware of the effects of mindless eating and reflecting on those in a conscious way.

Intuitive eating is a concept closely related to mindful eating. Principles of this way of eating include rejecting the dieting mentality, honoring one's hunger, and discovering one's satisfaction factor. Intuitive eating has three key components: unconditional permission to eat, eating for physical rather than emotional reasons, and relying on internal hunger, fullness, and satiety cues. If people eat intuitively, they remove the notion of "good" or "bad" foods and forbidden or permissible foods. This is thought to remove the emotions associated with food choice and self-judgment and results in food choices that provide sustenance and fuel rather than temporary feelings of comfort that soon turn to recrimination, regret, and self-criticism—feelings that may start a negative response and more emotional eating.

Intuitive eating has been studied as a way of mitigating problem eating and body image dissatisfaction (Bush, Rossy, Mintz, & Schopp, 2014). In this study, women and their partners who worked in a specific organization were enrolled in a 10-week study using the Eat for Life program. This program included weekly sessions where participants (n = 93) took part in a mindful meditation practice, a lecture on a topic related to intuitive eating, and discussion about the weekly homework assignments that participants were expected to complete. Homework assignments included reading the Eat for Life manual, daily guided meditation, and optional readings from a book titled *Breaking Free From Emotional Eating*. Compared to the wait-list control group (n = 100), participants in the intervention had better body appreciation, were more mindful, and ate more intuitively. They also were 3.65 times more likely to not show patterns of disordered eating.

STOP is another mindful eating method (Rubin, 2014). This four-bite method is thought to encourage mindful eating and helps people to pay attention to the first four bites of a meal.

1. **S**elect a bite of food carefully, imagining that you have never tasted this food before. Look carefully at all the food on your plate and then make your selection for this first bite.
2. **T**aste the food in your second bite by chewing slowly and noticing how the food changes as you chew.
3. **O**bserve how your hand moves to pick up the cutlery and then how it brings the food to your mouth. Also observe any feelings or thoughts as you enjoy your third bite of food.
4. **P**ause before you eat the fourth bite of food and pause again as you chew, before you swallow, and then again before you take your next bite of food.

These principles and actions are so different from the way that many of us and our patients eat. Many of us eat in front of the TV, at our desks, or on the run from one meeting or activity to the next. We barely have time to taste what we are eating and often do not even look at our plate until it is empty. Eating comprises bringing the fork or spoon to our mouths in a constant and repetitive movement, often not registering taste or texture, temperature, or appearance. We eat so quickly that we never realize when we are full or if we are still hungry. It takes 20 minutes for the brain to register satiety, but most of us consume what is in front of us in a much shorter time and eat until nothing is left rather than when our brain tells us we are satisfied and no longer hungry.

The Center for Mindful Eating (www.thecenterformindfuleating.org) is a not-for-profit organization that offers training and resources for individuals and professionals who practice this method. It has a registry of healthcare providers, mostly registered dietitians/nutritionists and psychotherapists but also nurses and physicians, from across the world.

Acceptance and Commitment Therapy

Another related concept is acceptance and commitment therapy (ACT) (Hayes, Levin, Plumb-Vilardaga, Villatte, & Pistorello, 2013). This is a relatively new model of behavior change that has components of mindfulness with the goal of encouraging the client (or patient) to enact behavior change that is congruent with personal values. ACT has six processes (Hayes, Luoma, Bond, Masuda, & Lillis, 2006):

1. Acceptance—This is an active and aware process of accepting what has happened or what the individual is feeling without judging or placing value on the event. It is the opposite of avoidance, an action that many people automatically turn to when they do not want to face something that is unpleasant or painful.
2. Cognitive diffusion—This is a technique where the individual is taught to change his or her response to negative thoughts.
3. Being present—By being present, the individual experiences the world more directly so that actions are more consistent with personal values.
4. Self as context—This refers to the individual being aware of his or her own history and experiences without attachment or investment so that acceptance occurs.
5. Values—The practitioner (usually a psychologist) helps the individual choose direction and action while actively ignoring negative messages or thoughts that might lead to avoidance or other nonproductive actions or behaviors.
6. Committed action—This is the final step, where the individual develops a way of behaving that is congruent with his or her values.

ACT was used in a study of 84 obese individuals who had completed at least six months of a weight-loss program (Lillis, Hayes, Bunting, & Masuda, 2009). Participants were randomized to either a one-day workshop using ACT principles or a wait-list group. Those in the intervention group showed greater decrease in feelings of stigma about their weight, were less distressed, had higher perceived quality of life, and lost more weight than the control group. Participants had better psychological health, even if they did not lose weight. The researchers concluded that the acceptance and value-based aspect of the intervention seemed to target avoidance and emotion-focused coping styles that are common in obese individuals who struggle to lose weight.

ACT also has been suggested as a useful way of helping those who have lost and regained weight. It may be used in conjunction with standard behavioral techniques as a precursor or add-on to more traditional weight-loss programs (Lillis & Kendra, 2014).

The Mindful Healthcare Provider

Lori Brotto, a practitioner and well-respected researcher in the area of mindfulness, suggests that in order to use mindfulness interventions with patients, we need to be mindful practitioners. She cautions that healthcare providers who attempt to teach mindfulness without being proficient in the practice will experience frustration and will not see results in their patients. The patients will experience the same frustration and lack of effectiveness (Brotto & Goldmeier, 2015). Multiple resources are available for healthcare providers and patients to learn and practice mindfulness. These are listed at the end of the chapter.

CASE VIGNETTE

C.W. is 72 years old and has been living with chronic lymphocytic lymphoma for 10 years. She is on a "watch-and-wait" regimen and has been doing well. She is happy that she has not had to have any active treatment thus far and would like to keep it that way. She is active in her community, plays bridge, and volunteers at the Humane Society. Her husband died six months ago, and although she appears to be dealing with his loss quite well, she has also gained some weight in the months since his death. She has come to the clinic for her regular appointment, and when she sees that she has gained five pounds, she bursts into tears. She admits that although her days are full, she is lonely at night and has been snacking while watching TV. She has never had to watch her weight before, but her clothes are feeling tight—and on her restricted budget, she does not want to have to buy new clothes.

Questions

1. Is a five-pound weight gain over six months something for C.W. to be concerned about? Why or why not?
2. What are some of the factors that may be involved in her weight gain?
3. How should the healthcare provider address this issue with an upset patient?

Using the NURSE method as described in Chapter 7, the healthcare provider can attempt to address some of the issues that C.W. may want to discuss.

Naming—"What is it about your weight today that has you so upset?"

Understanding—"Is it the weight gain alone or a combination of factors that is making you so upset? I wonder if this is somehow connected to the loss of your husband recently?"

Respecting—"I know this is something you might not want to talk about right now, but your emotional status is important for your overall health, and I would really like to offer you some help."

Supporting—"It must be lonely for you without your husband, especially at night. Many women tell me that the nighttime is the worst. That's when they turn to food to pass the time and make them feel less lonely. But snacking late at night can mean weight gain. Can we talk about this a little more after you've seen the doctor?"

Exploring—"Do you think that when you snack, you are fully aware of what you are eating? Often, eating in front of the TV uses just your mouth and not your brain. Do you know what I mean by that? One of the ways of dealing with this is to pay attention to what you are eating in a very intentional way. I am not saying that you cannot eat snacks in the evening, just that you can do so while paying attention to what you are eating and experiencing rather than just putting food in your mouth while your attention is on the TV. I have some books about this if you are interested."

Conclusion

Although not everyone is interested in a more cerebral approach to managing weight, increasing evidence supports that a more mindful approach to eating and weight loss can be helpful. Much like keeping to a diet and exercise regimen, being mindful and practicing mindfulness requires consistency and effort. Some individuals may find a combined approach of lifestyle change (diet and exercise) with mindfulness-based approaches to be effective.

Resources

Books

Bays, J.C. (2009). *Mindful eating: A guide to rediscovering a healthy and joyful relationship with food.* Boston, MA: Shambhala Publications.

Kabat-Zinn, J. (2005). *Guided mindfulness meditation: A complete guided mindfulness meditation program from Jon Kabat-Zinn.* Louisville, CO: Sounds True.

Kabat-Zinn, J. (2005). *Wherever you go, there you are.* New York, NY: Hachette Book Group.

Kabat-Zinn, J. (2011). *Mindfulness for beginners: Reclaiming the present moment—and your life*. Louisville, CO: Sounds True.

Puddicombe, A. (2012). *Get some headspace: How mindfulness can change your life in ten minutes a day*. New York, NY: St. Martin's Press.

Williams, M., & Penman, D. (2012). *Mindfulness: An eight-week plan for finding peace in a frantic world*. New York, NY: Rodale.

Additional Resources

- Headspace (www.headspace.com/andy-puddicombe): A meditation app where users can download sessions to their smartphones or tablets
- Jon Kabat-Zinn has a number of guided meditation CDs that range in experience level (from beginner to advanced). All are available at www.mindfulnesscds.com.
- The Mindfulness App: Meditation for Everyone (https://itunes.apple.com/us/app/mindfulness-app-meditation/id417071430?mt=8): An app by MindApps for iPhone users that provides guided meditation by Catherine Polan Orzech
- Mindfulness Meditation™ (www.mentalworkout.com/store/programs/mindfulness-meditation): An app by Mental Workout that provides instructions, exercises, and guided meditations by Stephan Bodian
- Additional meditation apps that are compatible with most smartphones are also available.

References

Alberts, H.J., Mulkens, S., Smeets, M., & Thewissen, R. (2010). Coping with food cravings: Investigating the potential of a mindfulness-based intervention. *Appetite, 55,* 160–163. doi:10.1016/j.appet.2010.05.044

Beshara, M., Hutchinson, A.D., & Wilson, C. (2013). Does mindfulness matter? Everyday mindfulness, mindful eating and self-reported serving size of energy dense foods among a sample of South Australian adults. *Appetite, 67,* 25–29. doi:10.1016/j.appet.2013.03.012

Brotto, L.A., & Goldmeier, D. (2015). Mindfulness interventions for treating sexual dysfunctions: The gentle science of finding focus in a multitask world. *Journal of Sexual Medicine, 12,* 1687–1689. doi:10.1111/jsm.12941

Bush, H.E., Rossy, L., Mintz, L.B., & Schopp, L. (2014). Eat for Life: A work site feasibility study of a novel mindfulness-based intuitive eating intervention. *American Journal of Health Promotion, 28,* 380–388. doi:10.4278/ajhp.120404-QUAN-186

Carmody, J.F., Olendzki, B.C., Merriam, P.A., Liu, Q., Qiao, Y., & Ma, Y. (2012). A novel measure of dietary change in a prostate cancer dietary program incorporating mindfulness training. *Journal of the Academy of Nutrition and Dietetics, 112,* 1822–1827. doi:10.1016/j.jand.2012.06.008

Cramer, H., Lauche, R., Paul, A., & Dobos, G. (2012). Mindfulness-based stress reduction for breast cancer—A systematic review and meta-analysis. *Current Oncology, 19,* e343–e352. doi:10.3747/co.19.1016

Dalen, J., Smith, B.W., Shelley, B.M., Sloan, A.L., Leahigh, L., & Begay, D. (2010). Pilot study: Mindful Eating and Living (MEAL): Weight, eating behavior, and psychological outcomes associated with a mindfulness-based intervention for people with obesity. *Complementary Therapies in Medicine, 18,* 260–264. doi:10.1016/j.ctim.2010.09.008

Daubenmier, J., Kristeller, J., Hecht, F.M., Maninger, N., Kuwata, M., Jhaveri, K., … Epel, E. (2011). Mindfulness intervention for stress eating to reduce cortisol and abdominal fat among overweight and obese women: An exploratory randomized controlled study. *Journal of Obesity, 2011,* 1–13. doi:10.1155/2011/651936

Gotink, R.A., Chu, P., Busschbach, J.J., Benson, H., Fricchione, G.L., & Hunink, M.G. (2015). Standardised mindfulness-based interventions in healthcare: An overview of systematic reviews and meta-analyses of RCTs. *PLOS ONE, 10,* e0124344. doi:10.1371/journal.pone.0124344

Hayes, S.C., Levin, M.E., Plumb-Vilardaga, J., Villatte, J.L., & Pistorello, J. (2013). Acceptance and commitment therapy and contextual behavioral science: Examining the progress of a distinctive model of behavioral and cognitive therapy. *Behavior Therapy, 44,* 180–198. doi:10.1016/j.beth.2009.08.002

Hayes, S.C., Luoma, J.B., Bond, F.W., Masuda, A., & Lillis, J. (2006). Acceptance and Commitment Therapy: Model, processes and outcomes. *Behavior Research and Therapy, 44,* 1–25. doi:10.1016/j.brat.2005.06.006

Huang, H.-P., He, M., Wang, H.-Y., & Zhou, M. (2016). A meta-analysis of the benefits of mindfulness-based stress reduction (MBSR) on psychological function among breast cancer (BC) survivors. *Breast Cancer, 23,* 568–576. doi:10.1007/s12282-015-0604-0

Jacobs, J., Cardaciotto, L., Block-Lerner, J., & McMahon, C. (2013). A pilot study of a single-session training to promote mindful eating. *Advances in Mind-Body Medicine, 27,* 18–23.

Kidd, L.I., Graor, C.H., & Murrock, C.J. (2013). A mindful eating group intervention for obese women: A mixed methods feasibility study. *Archives of Psychiatric Nursing, 27,* 211–218. doi:10.1016/j.apnu.2013.05.004

Lengacher, C.A., Reich, R.R., Kip, K.E., Barta, M., Ramesar, S., Paterson, C.L., … Park, J.Y. (2014). Influence of mindfulness-based stress reduction (MBSR) on telomerase activity in women with breast cancer (BC). *Biological Research for Nursing, 16,* 438–447. doi:10.1177/1099800413519495

Lillis, J., Hayes, S., Bunting, K., & Masuda, A. (2009). Teaching acceptance and mindfulness to improve the lives of the obese: A preliminary test of a theoretical model. *Annals of Behavioral Medicine, 37,* 58–69. doi:10.1007/s12160-009-9083-x

Lillis, J., & Kendra, K.E. (2014). Acceptance and Commitment Therapy for weight control: Model, evidence, and future directions. *Journal of Contextual Behavioral Science, 3,* 1–7. doi:10.1016/j.jcbs.2013.11.005

Ludwig, D., & Kabat-Zinn, J. (2008). Mindfulness in medicine. *JAMA, 300,* 1350–1352. doi:10.1001/jama.300.11.1350

Mantzios, M., & Wilson, J.C. (2013). Making concrete construals mindful: A novel approach for developing mindfulness and self-compassion to assist weight loss. *Psychology and Health, 29,* 422–441. doi:10.1080/08870446.2013.863883

Mathieu, J. (2009). What should you know about mindful and intuitive eating? *Journal of the American Dietetic Association, 109,* 1982–1987. doi:10.1016/j.jada.2009.10.023

Musial, F., Büssing, A., Heusser, P., Choi, K.-E., & Ostermann, T. (2011). Mindfulness-based stress reduction for integrative cancer care—A summary of evidence. *Forschende Komplementärmedizin, 18,* 192–202. doi:10.1159/000330714

O'Reilly, G.A., Cook, L., Spruijt-Metz, D., & Black, D.S. (2014). Mindfulness-based interventions for obesity-related eating behaviours: A literature review. *Obesity Reviews, 15,* 453–461. doi:10.1111/obr.12156

Papies, E.K., Pronk, T.M., Keesman, M., & Barsalou, L.W. (2015). The benefits of simply observing: Mindful attention modulates the link between motivation and behavior. *Journal of Personality and Social Psychology, 108,* 148–170. doi:10.1037/a0038032

Paulson, S., Davidson, R., Jha, A., & Kabat-Zinn, J. (2013). Becoming conscious: The science of mindfulness. *Annals of the New York Academy of Sciences, 1303,* 87–104. doi:10.1111/nyas.12203

Rouleau, C.R., Garland, S.N., & Carlson, L.E. (2015). The impact of mindfulness-based interventions on symptom burden, positive psychological outcomes, and biomarkers in cancer patients. *Cancer Management and Research, 7,* 121–131. doi:10.2147/CMAR.S64165

Rubin, R.C. (2014). The benefits of mindful eating. *Diabetes Self-Management, 31,* 20, 22–25.

Wansink, B., Painter, J.E., & North, J. (2005). Bottomless bowls: Why visual cues of portion size may influence intake. *Obesity Research, 13,* 93–100. doi:10.1038/oby.2005.12

Chapter 10
Challenges Faced by Patients Who Want to Lose Weight

Despite their best efforts, individuals who are overweight or obese may find it difficult to lose weight because of multiple factors. They may be emotional eaters with a lifetime of disordered eating in response to stress and negative emotions. Or, their families and friends may do their very best to sabotage their efforts to lose weight, most often from concerns about involuntary weight loss due to the cancer. They may initially lose weight but then gain it back over time. Whatever the reason, oncology care providers need to know and understand why it is so difficult for patients to do what seems best for themselves in this area, in part to be able to help patients overcome these barriers and also in an effort to support them through a challenging time.

It also is important for healthcare providers to recognize that we react to certain patients in less than optimal ways, and these "difficult" patients may provoke us to act in a way that is not therapeutic. Helping and encouraging patients to make lifestyle changes is an especially challenging area of health care, and we may encounter the greatest resistance in these situations. Learning to deal with patients who do not want to change can be challenging for many of us.

Emotional Eating

Emotional eating refers to the ingestion of food, often high-sugar, high-fat, or comfort foods, in response to stress or negative emotions. It is suggested that some individuals react to feeling sad or angry (both negative emotions) with a maladaptive response leading to overeating (Evers, Stok, & de Ridder, 2010). People who try to suppress their emotions in response to a stressor often eat more when negative emotions are present. Depression is known to be associated with emotional eating, as is post-traumatic stress disorder (PTSD) (Ouwens, van Strien, & van Leeuwe, 2009; Talbot, Maguen, Epel, Metzler, & Neylan, 2013). It is well documented that some cancer survivors experience symptoms suggestive of PTSD

(Shand, Cowlishaw, Brooker, Burney, & Ricciardelli, 2015). It is theorized that overeating at times of stress may temporarily reduce negative feelings (Dingemans, Martijn, Jansen, & van Furth, 2009), and individuals who tend to binge eat (eating large quantities of food at one time) also are more likely to be emotional eaters (Ricca et al., 2009). People who show negative coping styles are also those who tend to be emotional eaters. They tend to eat more when dealing with stress, and they may not be able to see themselves as able to cope with stress without engaging in emotional eating (Andrews, Lowe, & Clair, 2011). Food may be used as a distraction from stressful situations and a way of self-soothing (Hernandez-Hons & Woolley, 2012). Individuals who are trying to lose weight (termed *restrained eaters*) may also increase their intake of food when under stress or in response to positive emotions; the theory for this is that positive or negative emotions serve as a cognitive distraction for those trying to limit their food intake. They lose control of their ability to restrict their intake as a result (Macht, 2008).

Although no evidence exists in the literature about emotional eating in cancer survivors, it may be a coping mechanism used by cancer survivors, especially those who had a tendency to emotionally eat before their diagnosis. The cancer experience, from diagnosis through treatment and beyond, is highly traumatic for many, and dealing with the trauma through the use of previous and ingrained responses, including eating to soothe, distract, and counteract negative feelings, makes sense. Trying to change these responses may be almost impossible, and telling overweight or obese survivors to change their eating patterns in the face of the trauma of diagnosis and treatment is likely to be futile. It may be more effective to deal with the negative emotions that lead to emotional eating and encourage more effective coping mechanisms. This approach was used in a small study of mostly African American women who were overweight and self-reported to be emotional eaters (N = 79) (Goldbacher, La Grotte, Komaroff, Vander Veur, & Foster, 2015); no differences were found in outcomes.

How to Help Emotional Eaters

Temptation often plays a role in emotional eating. Most lapses in healthy eating are precipitated by temptation to eat food that either comforts or reduces stress. These high-fat and high-sugar foods often supply immediate gratification and a pleasurable sensory experience. "Liking" these kinds of food is one of the sentinel phenomena in the reward system that regulates eating. "Wanting" is the other phenomenon and is the process by which motivation, craving, and temptation occur (Appelhans, French, Pagoto, & Sherwood, 2016).

In a study of reasons why overweight and obese individuals eat unhealthy snacks, 55% reported that they ate these kinds of snacks because they looked or smelled tempting. About half (49%) said that they snacked because they were hungry, and 22% said that they snacked to ward off future hunger. Emotional eating happened in 10%–19% of respondents (Cleobury & Tapper, 2014).

Behavior therapy can be useful in teaching patients how to evaluate the events or cues that precipitate problem behaviors such as emotional eating. Helping patients to map out the events or feelings that lead to emotional eating can identify and address the sources of the problem (Kushner, Lawrence, & Kumar, 2013). When people are tempted by food or feel hungry and it is difficult for them to make rational choices, they are said to be in a "hot" state. The immediate reward or gratification of eating overrides their ability to think about the costs of eating unhealthy food. Trying to avoid unhealthy eating requires resistance to temptation. This can be done through having willpower, allowing the urge to pass, by deliberately ignoring the craving, or through cognitive restructuring or reappraisal (Appelhans et al., 2016).

Cognitive restructuring aims to limit the negative messages that overweight people often tell themselves when they eat something they should avoid. An example of a negative thought is: "I've blown it now by eating that cookie. I might as well just eat what I want for the rest of the day and start on my diet again tomorrow." Learning to think differently about small lapses stops that kind of catastrophic thinking and helps patients to see a lapse as a small bump in the road that can be overcome without losing control. A method to restructure the catastrophic thinking to something less negative is: "So, I ate a cookie . . . that does not mean I have ruined all the effort I have put into eating healthily this week. I am going to put that out of my mind, not beat myself up, and keep up the good progress I have made" (Kushner et al., 2013).

Another way of dealing with temptation is to prevent it from happening through controlling the environment and managing the stimulus to eat. Stimulus control helps patients manage the cues that drive them to eat. The sight and smell of food are powerful stimuli, and by controlling where and when they eat, patients can start to control their intake of food, particularly food that is not healthy for them. Three key principles for controlling stimuli include limiting where eating takes place (for example, only in the kitchen and dining room and not in front of the TV or computer), eating at regular times only, and not doing other activities while eating (for example, driving in the car or at the movies) (Kushner et al., 2013). These strategies involve executive function including working memory and cognitive flexibility. Working memory involves being able to recall and manipulate one's thoughts about food and what one needs to do to inhibit impulses to eat. Cognitive flexibility requires telling oneself that immediate gratification of the temptation will have negative results in the future. Both strategies are known to fail when a person is hungry and feeling negative emotions and fatigue (Appelhans et al., 2016).

Controlling the environment is not simple. When under the influence of their emotions, many people are able to find a way to find the food that they are craving—no matter what strategies they have used to control their environment. Commitment strategies involve restraining behavior by placing strict conditions around the activity, such as locking up tempting foods and allowing access to them only after an extended delay—at which point the craving may have passed.

Commitment by punishment is another strategy that has been tested. This involves some sort of negative consequence if the person fails to meet some predetermined goal. The punishment may be loss of money or some other desirable object. Social contracting with family and friends is another form of commitment. Commitment strategies are deemed more effective; however, they may not be easy to do (Appelhans et al., 2016). By publicly committing to some sort of behavior or goal, the loss of face and embarrassment of failing to keep the commitment may be effective for some. This is one of the principles of commercial weight-loss programs such as Weight Watchers, where public disclosure of weight gain (or loss) serves as a powerful social motivator.

Being able to control one's impulses may have more to do with personality traits than with cognition. People with high self-control traits are able to resist impulses and temptation far better than those with low self-control (Ent, Baumeister, & Tice, 2015). Willpower, being able to deal with temptation, is a cognitive function, and it is not possible to employ one's willpower at all times. Failure or giving in to temptation happens to many people, especially when their resistance to temptation is low (such as when they are tired, depressed, or stressed). An alternative to resisting temptation is to avoid it; however, this also is an act of self-control because avoidance requires planning and forethought as well as knowledge about oneself.

Maintaining Weight Loss

It is well known that most people who initially lose weight by following a diet and exercise regimen will eventually gain all or some of the weight back and may stop exercising as well. The National Institutes of Health have called for innovative strategies to address this issue (MacLean et al., 2015). They note that initially, patients will lose up to 8% of their body weight using traditional behavioral interventions, usually within the first six months. After that, patients tend to gain back two to four pounds per year. They theorize that this is because the costs of adherence to whatever intervention is being used exceed the perceived benefits of the weight loss. Initially, the benefits of adherence, such as clothes fitting better and receiving positive feedback from social contacts, is enough to maintain adherence. However, when maintaining weight loss is the goal, the positive feedback is outweighed by the effort that it takes to continue with the regimen. Another theory is that the original behaviors that caused weight gain in the first place comprise a set of eating habits. These are able to be controlled for a period of time. Eventually, however, these old habits return and the new way of eating, or rather controlling food intake, is subsumed.

Although these psychological theories may explain part of weight gain after initial weight loss, physiologic factors also may impede continued weight loss and cause weight gain. These factors include a negative energy balance and reduced energy stores. The body then maintains homeostasis by enhancing the reward mechanism for eating and diminishing the feeling of satiety, leading to overeating. Loss of lean tissue and reduced physical activity lead to a decline in metabolism, which further prompts weight gain.

How to Help Patients Maintain Weight Loss

Acceptance and commitment therapy (ACT), as discussed in Chapter 9, is suggested as a way to control challenges to self-regulation, which are seen as a threat to weight loss and weight-loss maintenance as well as engagement in physical activity. ACT uses a specific skill set to enable individuals to control weight. The first skill is a focus on personal values ("I want to be healthy so that I can play with my grandchildren"). Mindfulness and acceptance are skills that increase the commitment to value-based behavior (Lillis & Kendra, 2014).

Forman and Burtyn (2015) suggested that in today's world, an intrinsic drive to eat high-calorie foods occurs because these foods are so easily available. We do little physical activity because we have cars and elevators, so we are not required to expend a lot of physical energy. Therefore, overeating and being sedentary are default positions for many of us. The authors suggested that the difficulties many people experience in adhering to good eating and activity recommendations are due to an inability to control ourselves in the face of internal and external cues. They further suggested that successful control of weight is dependent on specific skills:

1. Knowing our personal values and committing to value-based behaviors
2. Awareness of higher-order thinking (metacognitive awareness)
3. Our ability to tolerate distress and reduction in pleasure

If our default setting is to not make good food choices and to participate in mostly sedentary behavior, it takes will and attention to make better choices. Given our natural tendencies and cues from the environment, focusing on something greater, such as personal values, becomes the motivation to make better choices (Forman & Burtyn, 2015). For the cancer survivor, this may be wanting to prevent recurrence or to live as long as possible to see children or grandchildren grow up. These value-based goals are seen as more motivating than losing weight merely to look better. It is important for people to be able to self-regulate their behavior. In the context of ACT, this means aligning current behavior ("I really want to eat that chocolate bar") with core values ("I want to be around to see my daughter get married"). It is suggested that not making the connection between values and behaviors results in mindless eating and avoidance of physical activity.

The third skill, being able to tolerate distress and reduction in pleasure, refers to our ability to respond to distressing emotions and feelings of hunger or food cravings in a constructive manner and not by giving in and eating to reduce the feelings in the moment. These feelings are generally experienced as aversive, but how we respond to them differs. Some people use distraction or suppression to deal with them, while others do something to change the experience. Successful self-control is not just being able to tolerate distress or upsetting situations but also being able to accept that something (for example, exercise) is not going to be immediately pleasurable (it may cause one to be short of breath, sweaty, and tired) and may not be as easy as sitting on the couch and watching TV.

Individuals who are stressed, fatigued, or anxious may find it difficult to deal with the emotional cues that drive them to overeat or avoid exercise. These individuals may need additional support to enable them to think about the values they hold for being healthy. They may also need encouragement to deal with the feelings they have that are making them want to overeat or avoid exercise.

Sabotage by Family and Friends

It is not uncommon for family and friends to try and sabotage the patient's weight loss. They may do this for a number of reasons: jealousy, guilt, concern for the patient's well-being, being misinformed about weight loss or gain in the context of cancer, or because the patient no longer wants to do things with family or friends that center around food. When the patient loses weight, people may feel threatened. Spouses may worry that their newly thin partner will leave them for someone more attractive. Family members may feel that the patient is judging them and their body habitus. Coworkers may interpret weight loss as a threat and think that the patient is going to be more successful than they are.

Sabotage can involve comments that are hurtful or deliberate attempts to tempt the patient who has lost weight into old eating patterns. Comments such as "You're not fun anymore now that you've lost weight" can be insulting and may make the patient feel isolated and guilty. Creating fear, whether out of genuine concern or due to lack of valid information, can be particularly stressful for the patient. Family members or friends may try to sabotage the patient's weight-loss efforts by implying that the patient's health will suffer if he or she gets "too thin." This may be a matter of an erroneous belief about cancer-related weight loss but also can be an emotionally coercive strategy to derail the patient's weight-loss efforts.

The following are some suggestions for responses that can be discussed with patients who are experiencing sabotage of their weight-loss efforts.

Comment 1: Are you sure you aren't getting too thin? You need to have some meat on your bones to withstand your treatment.

Response: Being overweight increases my risk of the cancer coming back. I've lost this weight on the advice of my healthcare providers, and they assure me that it is perfectly safe.

Comment 2: It won't hurt to have just one little piece of cake. It's my birthday, and I want you to celebrate it with me.

Response: One little piece of cake will lead to me eating way more than I need to or want. I am so happy to be here with you, and cake is not going to make the celebration any better.

Comment 3: I'm only doing this (bringing candy or other unhealthy snacks home) because I love you and am worried about you.

Response: I know you love me and are worried about me, but I would much rather have you go for a walk with me than tempt me with snacks.

Comment 4: You used to be so much more fun when you were drinking!

Response: I understand that it might feel that way to you, but without alcohol, I really am the real me, and I want to spend time with you being the real me, not someone who needs to be under the influence of alcohol to be "fun."

Although no single response can cover the many ways in which family and friends may sabotage weight loss in patients, it is important for patients to recognize when and how this happens and be prepared to deal with comments and attempts to derail their best efforts. Healthcare providers can help patients by raising the topic and providing anticipatory guidance to help them deal with a difficult situation that they may not have been expecting. Although some family members and friends will be supportive and celebratory of weight-loss success, others may not be able to.

Dealing With "Difficult" Patients

It is not uncommon for healthcare providers to find themselves with patients who are described as being "difficult." They may not listen to advice or follow prescriptions for healthy living. They may be argumentative or defensive (e.g., people who say "Yes, but . . ." in response to suggestions from their healthcare providers). They may be anxious or demanding, helpless, or "hopeless." These patients often elicit responses in their healthcare providers that we are not proud of. We may feel frustrated or angry and experience feelings of dread when we see the patient's name on our appointment list for the day.

Encouraging patients to make lifestyle changes is difficult, as making the changes is in itself difficult. Healthcare providers may feel useless when they have explained over and over why it is important for their patients to lose weight or start exercising. The temptation to just give up and not address these topics may be overwhelming. However, the golden moment when our patients finally "get it" and are ready to make the necessary changes may be at the next appointment or the one after that. Giving up is reflective of one's own frustration and not what our patients need.

Difficulties in patient encounters usually are related to problems with communication and may be patient, provider, or systems related (Breen & Greenberg, 2010; Lorenzetti, Jacques, Donovan, Cottrell, & Buck, 2013). Healthcare provider factors include poor communication skills, negative bias toward a certain kind of patient or certain patient conditions, and situational stressors. Patient factors include mental health issues, self-destructive behaviors, multiple and poorly defined symptoms or problems, and nonadherence to professional advice. Systems factors include lack of time and privacy, conflict with patients, and complex social issues that are difficult to deal with during busy clinic hours.

Suggestions for dealing with these difficult patients focus mostly on the healthcare provider in an attempt to reduce judgment and increase empathy. Mindfulness techniques, such as being consciously and intentionally attentive and present for the patient, have been shown to be useful to physicians (Sanyer & Fortenberry, 2013).

The Four Habits model has also been shown to be helpful (Stein, Frankel, & Krupat, 2005). These habits mirror many of the communication models described in Chapter 7 and illustrated throughout this book:

1. Being invested in the beginning by creating rapport quickly, finding out the patient's concerns, and planning the visit with the patient
2. Eliciting the patient's perspective by asking for any ideas about what is happening, determining the patient's goal for the visit, and exploring the effect of the symptom or illness on the patient's life
3. Demonstrating empathy by being open to the patient's emotions and conveying empathy both verbally and nonverbally
4. Investing in the end by delivering information, providing education, involving the patient in decision making, and summarizing the visit and discussing next steps

Other techniques include the BREATHE OUT intervention (Edgoose, Regner, & Zakletskaia, 2015) and the CALMER approach (Pomm, Shahady, & Pomm, 2004).

The BREATHE OUT approach is a two-step process. Before the visit, the healthcare provider should:

- List one **B**ias held about the patient.
- **RE**flect on why this patient is "difficult."
- List one thing to **A**ccomplish at the visit.
- **TH**ink about a question you would like to ask to explore the assumptions you hold.
- Stop before **E**ntering the patient's room and take three slow in-and-out breaths.

After the visit, the healthcare provider should:

- Reflect on the **O**utcome of the visit.
- Was anything **U**nexpected learned?
- Name one thing you would like to address with the patient **T**omorrow.

The CALMER approach contains the following:

- **C**atalyst for change
- **A**lter thoughts to change feelings.
- **L**isten and then make a diagnosis.
- **M**ake an agreement.
- **E**ducation and follow-up
- **R**each out and discuss feelings.

Catalyst for change refers to the fact that the patient is responsible for any changes in his or her life. Although healthcare providers cannot be responsible for any changes, they can control their own reactions to their patient and try to be helpful. **Altering thoughts to change feelings** describes the need for healthcare providers to consider the feelings elicited by their patient and how this might be affecting the patient–provider relationship. **Listen and then make a diagnosis** puts the emphasis on being attentive to what the patient is saying and only then making a diagnosis or decision about what comes next. By **making an agreement** with the patient to continue with the therapeutic relationship, both the patient and provider come to the understanding that they have made a conscious decision to continue working together to solve the patient's problems. **Education and follow-up** should be offered based on the needs and readiness for change of the patient and not on the provider's agenda. Finally, the provider is encouraged to **reach out** for support from colleagues to help deal with any residual feelings of frustration or distress they have from the patient encounter.

CASE VIGNETTE

J.T. is a 62-year-old man with advanced prostate cancer who has struggled to lose weight after gaining 30 pounds while on androgen deprivation therapy. He admits that he is depressed and finds the evenings particularly bad, as he lives alone and tends to eat cookies, cakes, and ice cream (all of which he buys for his grandchildren who visit on the weekends) after dinner while watching TV. Despite seeing a nutritionist regularly, his weight continues to climb, and he is noticeably short of breath when he walks into your office. Using the SPIKES format (see Chapter 7), how would you incorporate the principles discussed in this chapter in supporting J.T.?

Setting

Choose a setting that is private and where disturbances are minimized, as you would with any discussion where the content is potentially sensitive or likely to evoke an emotional response. Avoid distractions and focus on the patient in a calm and engaged manner.

Perception

Nurse: It seems to me like you are really struggling to lose the weight you've gained during treatment. What do you think is going on?

J.T.: Well, I've always been a "sweets" person. I love anything with chocolate or cream. Since my wife passed, it's been really difficult. The nights are so long, and I miss her something fierce. So, I eat.

Invitation or Information

Nurse: I hear you. Loneliness is a powerful temptation to eat food, especially comfort food, and you seem to especially like food that is not going to help you lose weight. I know you've seen a nutritionist, but you don't seem to be getting a handle on this. Have you talked to her about doing something to get control over your cravings?

J.T.: I'm not sure that the nutritionist is helpful at all. She keeps giving me books to read and stuff like that, and I really am trying, but nothing seems to help.

Knowledge

Nurse: We know that losing weight is difficult—and for some of us, it feels like it's impossible. It's also really hard when the treatment you are having seems to add the pounds without much effort on your part. But we know that there are powerful motivators that help us to keep trying. You seem so connected to your grandchildren. What are your hopes and dreams for them and your relationship with them?

J.T.: Oh, yes! I do love those kids, especially the oldest—My Little Princess, I call her. Ellie is 10 going on 21, and we just love to watch TV together. And of course I love the others, too. There's Brad, who's 6, and the baby, Oliver, who just turned 4. I love them all to bits, and really, I live for the weekends when they come over to see me.

Nurse: So, watching them grow up and being a part of their future is important to you. That can be a powerful motivator to help you be healthy.

J.T.: I never thought of it that way. If I want to be around to see Ellie married, well, I'd need to watch myself, right?

Empathy

Nurse: Lots of people find the nights really difficult, especially if they live alone. Chocolate and ice cream can be a comfort, but it only lasts a few seconds, right?

J.T.: You're right. Then the guilt sets in and then I find that I just can't stop because I've blown it, you know? So, I just keep on shoving the food into my mouth.

Summarize or Strategize

Nurse: So, let me summarize: Being part of your grandchildren's lives is important to you, and you want to be healthy so that you can be involved with them for a long time into the future. So, you have a reason to be motivated to be as healthy as you can be. However, you are at times lonely, especially at night, and you find yourself eating comfort food to help you deal with your emotions. I know that we can work with this and help find you some ways of coping with your feelings, and that, in turn, will help you find other ways to deal with your emotions. Are you ready to do some work on this?

J.T.: I'll try anything because what I'm doing obviously isn't working. So, what do you think I can do?

Conclusion

Most cancer survivors want to do the very best they can to get well, prevent recurrence, and live a full and healthy life. But life gets in the way, and they often revert to old habits and ways of being that counteract the best advice and guidance we give them. This chapter addressed some of the common challenges faced by those who want to lose weight or who have lost weight and then find themselves struggling to keep the weight off. Emotional eating and sabotage by family and friends are realities in the lives of our patients, and we need to support them in their efforts to deal with these challenges. Healthcare providers are, in essence, real people, and sometimes our patients push our buttons and frustrate and irritate us. We have to learn how to deal with these "difficult" patients because they are often the ones most in need of care.

References

Andrews, R.A., Lowe, R., & Clair, A. (2011). The relationship between basic need satisfaction and emotional eating in obesity. *Australian Journal of Psychology, 63,* 207–213. doi:10.1111/j.1742-9536.2011.00021.x

Appelhans, B.M., French, S.A., Pagoto, S.L., & Sherwood, N.E. (2016). Managing temptation in obesity treatment: A neurobehavioral model of intervention strategies. *Appetite, 96,* 268–279. doi:10.1016/j.appet.2015.09.035

Breen, K.J., & Greenberg, P.B. (2010). Difficult physician–patient encounters. *Internal Medicine Journal, 40,* 682–688. doi:10.1111/j.1445-5994.2010.02311.x

Cleobury, L., & Tapper, K. (2014). Reasons for eating 'unhealthy' snacks in overweight and obese males and females. *Journal of Human Nutrition and Dietetics, 27,* 333–341. doi:10.1111/jhn.12169

Dingemans, A.E., Martijn, C., Jansen, A.T.M., & van Furth, E.F. (2009). The effect of suppressing negative emotions on eating behavior in binge eating disorder. *Appetite, 52,* 51–57. doi:10.1016/j.appet.2008.08.004

Edgoose, J.Y., Regner, C.J., & Zakletskaia, L.I. (2015). BREATHE OUT: A randomized controlled trial of a structured intervention to improve clinician satisfaction with "difficult" visits. *Journal of the American Board of Family Medicine, 28,* 13–20. doi:10.3122/jabfm.2015.01.130323

Ent, M.R., Baumeister, R.F., & Tice, D.M. (2015). Trait self-control and the avoidance of temptation. *Personality and Individual Differences, 74,* 12–15. doi:10.1016/j.paid.2014.09.031

Evers, C., Stok, F.M., & de Ridder, D.T.D. (2010). Feeding your feelings: Emotion regulation strategies and emotional eating. *Personality and Social Psychology Bulletin, 36,* 792–804. doi:10.1177/0146167210371383

Forman, E.M., & Butryn, M.L. (2015). A new look at the science of weight control: How acceptance and commitment strategies can address the challenge of self-regulation. *Appetite, 84,* 171–180. doi:10.1016/j.appet.2014.10.004

Goldbacher, E., La Grotte, C., Komaroff, E., Vander Veur, S., & Foster, G.D. (2015). An initial evaluation of a weight loss intervention for individuals who engage in emotional eating. *Journal of Behavioral Medicine, 39,* 139–150. doi:10.1007/s10865-015-9678-6

Hernandez-Hons, A., & Woolley, S.R. (2012). Women's experiences with emotional eating and related attachment and sociocultural processes. *Journal of Marital and Family Therapy, 38,* 589–603. doi:10.1111/j.1752-0606.2011.00239.x

Kushner, R., Lawrence, V., & Kumar, S. (2013). *Practical manual of clinical obesity.* Hoboken, NJ: Wiley-Blackwell.

Lillis, J., & Kendra, K.E. (2014). Acceptance and Commitment Therapy for weight control: Model, evidence, and future directions. *Journal of Contextual Behavioral Science, 3,* 1–7. doi:10.1016/j.jcbs.2013.11.005

Lorenzetti, R.C., Jacques, C.H., Donovan, C., Cottrell, S., & Buck, J. (2013). Managing difficult encounters: Understanding physician, patient, and situational factors. *American Family Physician, 87,* 419–425.

Macht, M. (2008). How emotions affect eating: A five-way model. *Appetite, 50,* 1–11. doi:10.1016/j.appet.2007.07.002

MacLean, P.S., Wing, R.R., Davidson, T., Epstein, L., Goodpaster, B., Hall, K.D., … Ryan, D. (2015). NIH working group report: Innovative research to improve maintenance of weight loss. *Obesity, 23,* 7–15. doi:10.1002/oby.20967

Ouwens, M.A., van Strien, T., & van Leeuwe, J.F.J. (2009). Possible pathways between depression, emotional and external eating: A structural equation model. *Appetite, 53,* 245–248. doi:10.1016/j.appet.2009.06.001

Pomm, H., Shahady, E., & Pomm, R. (2004). The CALMER approach: Teaching learners six steps to serenity when dealing with difficult patients. *Family Medicine, 36,* 467–469.

Ricca, V., Castellini, G., Lo Sauro, C., Ravaldi, C., Lapi, F., Mannucci, E., … Faravelli, C. (2009). Correlations between binge eating and emotional eating in a sample of overweight subjects. *Appetite, 53,* 418–421. doi:10.1016/j.appet.2009.07.008

Sanyer, O.N., & Fortenberry, K. (2013). Using mindfulness techniques to improve difficult clinical encounters. *American Family Physician, 87,* 402.

Shand, L.K., Cowlishaw, S., Brooker, J.E., Burney, S., & Ricciardelli, L.A. (2015). Correlates of post-traumatic stress symptoms and growth in cancer patients: A systematic review and meta-analysis. *Psycho-Oncology, 24,* 624–634. doi:10.1002/pon.3719

Stein, T., Frankel, R.M., & Krupat, E. (2005). Enhancing clinician communication skills in a large healthcare organization: A longitudinal case study. *Patient Education and Counseling, 58,* 4–12. doi:10.1016/j.pec.2005.01.014

Talbot, L.S., Maguen, S., Epel, E.S., Metzler, T.J., & Neylan, T.C. (2013). Post-traumatic stress disorder is associated with emotional eating. *Journal of Traumatic Stress, 26,* 521–525. doi:10.1002/jts.21824

Chapter 11
Resources

A number of resources are available to oncology and other healthcare providers that provide guidance and assistance for those who want to learn more about managing obesity in their patients. Guidelines specific to cancer care in the context of overweight and obesity are beginning to be developed. This will no doubt continue to grow as the associations between overweight and obesity and cancer become more apparent and perhaps better accepted.

Academy of Nutrition and Dietetics

The Academy of Nutrition and Dietetics' website contains a wealth of information for the public and professionals about food, fitness, and health.

www.eatright.org

American Cancer Society

The American Cancer Society publishes nutrition and physical activity guidelines every five years. A summation of these recommendations for healthcare providers about nutrition and exercise for cancer survivors through all stages of the cancer continuum is available at http://onlinelibrary.wiley.com/doi/10.3322/caac.20140/full.

www.cancer.org

American College of Cardiology/American Heart Association

The American Heart Association published the *2013 AHA/ACC/TOS Guideline for the Management of Overweight and Obesity in Adults: A Report of the American College of Cardiology/American Heart Association Task Force on Practice Guidelines and the Obesity Society*, a guideline for primary care providers with patients who are overweight or obese. This comprehensive guideline has information that may be useful and can be applied to adults with cancer.

http://content.onlinejacc.org/article.aspx?articleid=1770219

American College of Sports Medicine

The American College of Sports Medicine Roundtable on Exercise Guidelines for Cancer Survivors advocates that survivors follow the 2008 U.S. Department of Health and Human Services recommendations for physical activity for all Americans, with adaptations based on disease- and treatment-related problems. Avoidance of inactivity is regarded as the most important recommendation even for those experiencing side effects from treatment.

http://journals.lww.com/acsm-msse/Fulltext/2010/07000/American_College_of_Sports_Medicine_Roundtable_on.23.aspx

American Society of Clinical Oncology

American Society of Clinical Oncology guidelines include reference to the American Cancer Society guidelines for nutrition and physical activity; the American College of Sports Medicine exercise guidelines for cancer survivors; the Centers for Disease Control and Prevention strategies for obesity prevention; and the National Heart, Lung, and Blood Institute (NHLBI) clinical guidelines on the identification, evaluation, and treatment of overweight and obesity in adults.

www.asco.org/practice-guidelines/cancer-care-initiatives/prevention-survivorship/obesity-cancer/obesity-clinical

Body Assessment Guidelines

Body mass index (BMI) is a way of assessing a person's weight to classify him or her as normal, underweight, overweight, or obese. It is calculated by dividing the person's weight (in kg or lb) by his or her height (in cm or in) (see Table 11-1). Additional information on BMIs is available at www.cdc.gov/healthyweight/assessing/bmi/adult_bmi/index.html.

Table 11-1. Standard Body Mass Index (BMI) Categorization

BMI	Weight Status
< 18.5	Underweight
18.5–24.9	Normal or healthy weight
25.0–29.9	Overweight
≥ 30.0	Obese

Note. From "About Adult BMI," by Centers for Disease Control and Prevention, 2015. Retrieved from https://www.cdc.gov/healthyweight/assessing/bmi/adult_bmi/index.html.

Additional ways to measure body fat include skinfold thickness and other more technical measures. BMI, however, is widely used, as it is easy to calculate with readily available tables.

A useful online BMI calculator is available at www.nhlbi.nih.gov/health/educational/lose_wt/BMI/bmicalc.htm.

Another measure of risk related to weight is the waist-to-hip ratio. Individuals with larger waist measurement are at greater risk of poor health than those with greater hip measurement.

- A ratio of 0.95 or below (men) or 0.80 or below (women) = low risk

- A ratio of 0.96–1.0 (men) or 0.81–0.85 (women) = moderate risk
- A ratio of more than 1.0 (men) or more than 0.85 (women) = high risk

An online calculator is available at www.bmi-calculator.net/waist-to-hip-ratio-calculator.

Centers for Disease Control and Prevention

The Centers for Disease Control and Prevention has a comprehensive list of strategies and guidelines related to obesity prevention, nutrition, and physical activity.

www.cdc.gov/obesity/resources/strategies-guidelines.html

National Comprehensive Cancer Network

The National Comprehensive Cancer Network® does not currently have a guideline specific to overweight and obesity; however, the need for attention to this topic is included in its survivorship guidelines, which is available at www.nccn.org/professionals/physician_gls/pdf/survivorship.pdf.

www.nccn.org

National Heart, Lung, and Blood Institute

NHLBI published federal guidelines in collaboration with the National Institutes of Health for the identification, assessment, and treatment of overweight and obesity. NHLBI published *Clinical Guidelines on the Identification, Evaluation, and Treatment of Overweight and Obesity in Adults: The Evidence Report*, a free downloadable e-book that contains evidence-based information on approaches to managing overweight and obesity in adults.

http://catalog.nhlbi.nih.gov/catalog/product/Clinical-Guidelines-on-the-Identification-Evaluation-and-Treatment-of-Overweight-and-Obesity-in-Adults-The-Evidence-Report/98-4083

Nutrition.gov

This federally sponsored website provides science-based information on a variety of topics related to healthy eating, fitness, and food safety.

www.nutrition.gov

Obesity Society

This professional organization supports research in obesity and education for the public and professionals, as well as advocacy for those with obesity. The society produces a professional journal, *Obesity*, which is accessible at www.obesity.org/publications/obesity-journal.

www.obesity.org

Oncology Nursing Society

The Oncology Nursing Society has an initiative developed by member experts to encourage oncology nurses to promote physical activity to patients during treatment. The initiative is called Get Up, Get Moving, and the website contains useful resources for oncology nurses, including a course to further educate nurses to become leaders in the field, evidence-based resources, a teaching video for use with patients, and a link to a quality measures registry.

www.ons.org/practice-resources/get-up-get-moving

U.S. Department of Agriculture

The U.S. Department of Agriculture has reliable dietary information and guidelines, including the 2015–2020 U.S. guidelines, and useful resources for healthcare providers.

http://choosemyplate.gov

Index

The letter *f* after a page number indicates that relevant content appears in a figure; the letter *t*, in a table.

C

D

E

F

N

O

P

R